Activating the Learner's Brain

Activating the Learner's Brain

Using the Learner's Brain Model

Dr. Mario C. Barbiere

ROWMAN & LITTLEFIELD
Lanham • Boulder • New York • London

Published by Rowman & Littlefield
A wholly owned subsidiary of The Rowman & Littlefield Publishing Group, Inc.
4501 Forbes Boulevard, Suite 200, Lanham, Maryland 20706
www.rowman.com

Unit A, Whitacre Mews, 26–34 Stannary Street, London SE11 4AB

Copyright © 2018 by Mario C. Barbiere

All rights reserved. No part of this book may be reproduced in any form or by any electronic or mechanical means, including information storage and retrieval systems, without written permission from the publisher, except by a reviewer who may quote passages in a review.

British Library Cataloguing in Publication Information Available

Library of Congress Cataloging-in-Publication Data Is Available
ISBN 978-1-4758-3720-9 (cloth: alk. paper)
ISBN 978-1-4758-3721-6 (pbk: alk. paper)
ISBN 978-1-4758-3722-3 (electronic)

This book is dedicated to the family: Jim, Mairin, Kaleb, and Kaia; Chris, Mike and Jackie; Matt; brothers Charlie and Ray; extended family: Jim and Diane, John and Pat, Janice and Mark, and Carol and Mark. Family is forever.

Contents

Preface		ix
Acknowledgments		xi
Introduction: A Summary of the Chapters		1
1	Lesson Delivery	5
2	Using Assessments	33
3	Consolidation for Closure	61
4	Reflections	73
5	Sample Lesson Plans: Putting It All Together	89
Appendix A: Rubric 1: Questioning		117
Appendix B: Rubric 2: Student Engagement		121
Appendix C: Rubric 3: Student Interviews		123
Appendix D: Rubric 4: Coaching Walkthrough Using the Learner's Brain Model		125
Index		131
About the Author		135

Preface

How many times has a teacher been asked: Is this going to be on the test? Why do we have to know this? When will I use this? Or how many times has a teacher wondered why students can play video games for hours but they have a hard time paying attention in class. One can hear teachers say: "Why doesn't the student get it, I taught the information and yet it seems like this is the first time that the student is seeing or hearing it." These kinds of questions get to the heart of the teaching and learning process.

When students ask the above "killer questions," they are asking questions that delve into the heart of the teaching-learning process. The meaning of the killer question is very simple: will this information be on a test? If it will not be on a test, then the student perceives that there is no value to the information. What the student is saying is that the information has no perceived value, but if it is going to be on the test, then the student should pay attention.

The question about "why do I have to know this" and "when will I use it" addresses the concerns students have that information has little or no merit or value. The students fail to see the application of information.

This book, *Activating the Learner's Brain*, addresses the questions stated earlier by providing strategies for delivering instruction that makes sense to the learner and has meaning. Making sense and having meaning are two important factors for information to become permanent.

The first chapter of the book discusses how the Learner's Brain Model uses right- and left-brain research for lesson design and why lessons need to incorporate the logical (left brain) and the global perspective (right brain) so students can move from the "informational" age to the "conceptual" age. The goal is to plan lessons so students can apply information and concepts to real-life problems. The focus is for teachers to use brain research about the learner so the lessons are more effective.

Delivering lessons focused on student interest will answer the question why students can play video games for hours. They can play video games for hours because they are interested in what they are doing so their attention is focused. The task is to promote the same interest in teacher lessons so as to focus student attention. Other variables that keep students interested in video games are the ability to set long- and short-term goals; video games are interactive, and immediate feedback is provided. Because the activity is adaptive, students build on their successes, and they move from success to success.

Subsequent chapters mirror the pluses of video games as teacher delivery must be adaptive throughout the instructional delivery so assessments are discussed following the chapter on instructional delivery. It is the value of assessments that teachers need to know so they can adapt to monitor their instructional delivery. The use of assessments and checks for understanding throughout the lesson is the feedback that the teacher receives from the student so the teacher can adapt his or her lesson. The more immediate the feedback, the more effective the instruction will be. The immediate feedback students get from playing a video game (blowing up or going back to the beginning) gives them a wealth of knowledge and allows them to adjust their strategies.

The value of feedback is not only during a lesson but at the end of the less. Accordingly, the next chapter after assessment is consolidation for close. It is the consolidation for closure that students give teachers that enables teachers to plan their next lesson. The text provides ways of doing closure overtly or covertly. Auditory, visual, kinesthetic, or tactile closure strategies are also provided. The various strategies address student's different learning styles and preferences.

The last chapter is devoted to reflection: just like the student who plays a video game and does not do well, the student reflects on what worked and what needs to be done when he or she plays again. Student reflection is necessary to promote self-regulation and self-monitoring of student work. Like the student who reflects on a video game, the teacher reflects on his or her lesson to determine what worked and what needs to be adjusted. Reflection is necessary for the teacher and the student.

To help teachers with the instructional process, rubrics are provided that can be used for teachers to coach themselves up or for administrators to use to coach teachers.

This book can be used for a book study, for teachers to use for assessing their own teaching, for administrators to use for coaching teachers, or for parents to use for helping their children regulate and monitor their learning. A field book with activities is available which can be a companion to this book.

Acknowledgments

Sometimes people see something in you that you don't see. My mother wanted her son to go to college and insisted that I take college prep courses in high school. She won that discussion. It was Mr. Massamino, the basketball coach, who suggested the college to this football player and so the journey began. My father was proud of me that I would be going to college. My mother always believed that i should go to college and now her dream was coming true.

My brothers, Charlie and Ray, made growing up fun and more importantly, taught me the value of family.

Seton Hall University made me a "believer" that one should dream big. Their doctoral program was challenging, but the professors were positive, compassionate, and supportive. I learned that "Believing is Seeing."

Doing the work of school turnaround has been exciting and personally rewarding. It was made rewarding by the spirit of cooperation from the teachers, assistant principals, supervisors, principals, central office administrators, and superintendents I worked with in the many counties in New Jersey.

Thank you, Carlie Wall and Tom Koerner, as well as Rowman & Littlefield for making my dream become a reality.

Finally, the teachers involved in school turnaround who believe and make student dreams come true, your efforts are acknowledged and appreciated. Believe in students, and they will "see" it and achieve success that we all want for our scholars. We never want to extinguish hope and dreams as that may be the only thing one has.

Introduction

A Summary of the Chapters

CHAPTER 1: LESSON DELIVERY

Focus of the Chapter

The informational stage involves providing teacher-directed instruction, student-directed instruction, independent work, small group activities, and/or cooperative activities. Strategies for each phase of the informational stage will be provided.

Introduction

How does the Learner's Brain Model use right- and left-brain research for lesson design? Why do lessons need the logical (left brain) and the global perspective (right brain) as educators move from the "informational" age to the "conceptual" age? How do we plan lessons applying information and concepts to real-life problems? Additionally, how can lessons be planned using brain research, and how does the learner process information so the lessons are more effective?

Probing Questions

1. How do I plan a lesson using brain research about the nature of the learner?
2. What is gradual release?
3. Competency versus performance?
4. How does the teacher pace the lesson?

CHAPTER 2: USING ASSESSMENTS

Focus of the Chapter

This chapter will focus on how to use assessments to make lessons successful, monitoring student progress using formative and summative assessments and using data to drive instruction. The focus of the chapter is on analyzing data so the teacher is not "data rich" and "analysis poor."

Introduction

Is testing the student or teacher's friend or foe? How can assessments be used for learning and not of learning? This chapter will discuss how assessments can determine what was effectively taught. Additionally, how assessments can be used for promoting long-term retention will be discussed.

Probing Questions

1. Are assessments for learning or of learning?
2. Masses or distributed learning?
3. How do I know if students are learning throughout the lesson?
4. How can I use visual, auditory, kinesthetic, or tactile checks of understanding to assess student learning?

CHAPTER 3: CONSOLIDATION FOR CLOSURE

Focus of the Chapter

The teacher will learn strategies to use for consolidation for closure. The teacher will also be able to show the students strategies they can use for self-regulation when doing home learning.

Introduction

Consolidation for closure is a process whereby the learner will summarize what has been learned. Although closure is usually done at the end of a lesson, it can be done during the lesson. What research says about closure and overt or covert closure strategies for visual, auditory, tactile, or kinesthetic learners will be provided.

Probing Questions

1. Why is consolidation for closure done?
2. How will the students show the teacher what they learned?

3. How will the teacher use what the students learned to plan the lesson for the next day?
4. Can overt or covert consolidation for closure use visual, auditory, kinesthetic, or tactile strategies?

CHAPTER 4: REFLECTIONS

Focus of the Chapter

This chapter will discuss research on reflection and provide strategies to use for reflection. How will students self-check their work, and what will they use for the reflective process? Rubrics will be provided for the process.

Introduction

This chapter will seek to answer the following questions: What is the value of reflection? How is reflection used in lesson design? Once the questions are answered, the students can self-check and self-modulate their work based on their reflection.

Probing Questions

1. What is the purpose of reflection?
2. Why is reflection necessary to empower teachers?
3. How can a teacher promote reflection for student self-regulation?
4. Why is reflection necessary to empower students?

CHAPTER 5: SAMPLE LESSON PLANS: PUTTING IT ALL TOGETHER

Focus of the Chapter

This chapter will provide sample lesson and break down each component of the lesson. Lessons for different grade levels will be provided.

Introduction

What does an effective lesson plan look like? More importantly, what is the research to ensure that the lesson is effective? Sample plans will provide a framework for teachers to see how the components of lesson design are needed for effective instructional delivery.

APPENDICES

Focus

The appendices will provide various rubrics referenced throughout the book that can be used for coaching or for self-evaluation. Teachers can use the rubrics for self-improvement, peer coaching, or self-assessment.

Introduction

The rubrics are provided for teachers or administrators to use for "coaching," for self-improvement and are tied to research so they can be used in conjunction with any evaluation system.

Chapter 1

Lesson Delivery

FOCUS OF THE CHAPTER

The informational stage of instruction is the "input" phase of the instructional process whereby the teacher provides the information to the student relative to the Student Learning Target. The teacher will construct the learning environment based on the learning target and can employ teacher-directed instruction, student-directed instruction, independent work, and/or cooperative activities to meet the learning target. Strategies for the various phases will be provided.

INTRODUCTION

As you read the chapter, ask yourself the questions noted as the questions will provide focus for the chapter. How does the Learner's Brain Model use right- and left-brain research for lesson design? Why do lessons need the logical (left brain) and the global perspective (right brain) as educators move from the "informational" age to the "conceptual" age? How do we plan lessons applying information and concepts to real-life problems? How can lessons be planned using brain research? The schema for lesson delivery is in Figure 1.3.

Probing Questions

1. How do I plan a lesson using brain research about the nature of the learner?
2. What is gradual release?
3. Competency versus performance?
4. How does the teacher pace the lesson?

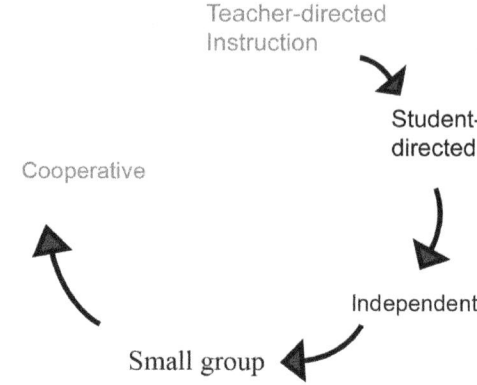

Figure 1.1

A schema of the instructional delivery phase of the Learner's Brain Model is Figure 1.1 Prior to beginning the instructional delivery phase of the Learner's Brain Model, the teacher should investigate the answers to the following questions:

- What prior knowledge do the students have regarding the subject/topic? Once this is determined, the instructor will decide what content will be taught, and how it will be delivered to the students. (Content question)
- What Common Core State Standards (CCSS), relative to the topic, will be my focus, and what objective(s) are needed to address the standard? (Curriculum alignment to standards-based instruction)
- What previous assessment data are available to use, and how do teachers use these data as a starting point for their instructional planning? (Use of assessments to plan and differentiate instruction)
- What is the learning outcome for students? (Student Learning Target) How will the teachers know that they learned what was taught? (Demonstration of Student Learning [DSL])
- What do the teachers expect their students to learn and recall by the end of the lesson? (Short-term goal for the development of the Student Learning Target (objective))
- How will I introduce the information, in order to motivate student interest and promote readiness? (What Readiness Set is needed to establish an effective emotional climate and activate prior knowledge?)
- What resources are necessary to accomplish strategic objectives and goals? (Implementation of resources is necessary in the teaching process.)
- How will the teachers evaluate student learning during and after the lesson? (Strategic checks for understanding/informal and formative assessments, and questioning techniques, are performed throughout the lesson.)

- How will the teachers conclude the lesson and apply their data collection to subsequent lessons? (Consolidation for closure activities)

CURRICULA DRIVE INSTRUCTIONAL DELIVERY

The above questions are essential to identify curricular components based on standards and instructional strategies to use. The curricula will drive the instructional delivery, please reference Figure 1.1 for a schema for delivery. The instructional delivery will drive the instructional strategies for the teacher to plan. Planning and evaluation of the lesson are paramount; hence, the critical questions for planning are: How will the teacher determine his or her starting point of the lesson? How will the teacher assess the student's prior knowledge of the subject matter?

The answers to these two questions lie in pre-assessment. Teachers often view an assessment as a test or quiz that comes at the end of a study unit, which determines and evaluates what students have learned. This process is consistent with the strategy of collecting summative data. The problem with summative data is that it is done at the end of a unit. Some folks would say that it is akin to doing an autopsy.

THE ROLE OF FORMATIVE ASSESSMENTS

Formative assessments are done throughout the learning experience like frequent wellness visits. They are checks along the way. In our twenty-first-century age of knowledge, we realize that today's assessment is tomorrow's instruction. Interpretation of the assessment(s) provides information to the teachers, regarding students' knowledge about the lesson and their mastery of the skills or concepts being taught. Once this information is secured, it can be used as the pivotal starting point for differentiated instruction since each student has individual levels or starting points.

Through the process of focusing on formative assessment to get student data, teachers see that differentiation is not a single planned event, but rather a process that occurs naturally when teachers set goals, observe the student progress to those goals, and then respond accordingly.

This process frames the teachers' mind-set, to the possibility, that differentiation could be part of their daily instruction, rather than a strategy reserved for large, cumulative projects. The action theory pertaining to the use of assessments for daily differentiated planning requires teachers to understand their cliental, to be able to self-motivate and facilitates the student's learning, and empowering the students in such a way that foundationally builds appropriate twenty-first-century learners and promotes a self-learning student working in a climate for learning.

Specifically, teachers are responding to the needs of their students based on assessment data. Assessment drives instruction. The quickest way to differentiate instruction is to use formative assessments that provide immediate information.

Normally, formative assessments are used throughout the lesson to collect data; however, the data collection process can also begin at the end of the previous lesson.

USING ASSESSMENT VIA CONSOLIDATION FOR CLOSURE

Teachers can conduct an assessment (Consolidation for Closure activity) at the end of the lesson, and the consolidation activity provides information to the teachers regarding the outcome of the lesson. The information can be developed and included in the subsequent lesson. A good example of this concept is the use of an "exit ticket."

An exit ticket activity is a reflective practice, which provides feedback to the teacher. It encourages the students to synthesize the newly learned information and recall it prior to leaving the class for the day. A teacher may say, "Tell me one thing you learn today or write down one thing that was confusing to you today."

CONSOLIDATION FOR CLOSURE "SUNNY POINT/ CLOUDY POINT"

A Consolidation for Closure activity is "Sunny Point/Cloudy Point." The Sunny Point is what students report they know, and the Cloudy Point is what they are confused. They write a Sunny Point and a Cloudy Point on an index card and give it to the teacher on the way out of class. The information gained by the teacher will be critical to planning the next day's lesson.

The use of an exit card or any other closure activity addresses the answer to the initial aforementioned question "what does the student know and how is it demonstrated to me?" Based upon the answer to this question, the teacher may consider reteaching aspects of the lesson or proceed with a new lesson.

After the data from the Consolidation for Closure activity is gathered and reviewed by the teacher, the teacher can assess the student progress for future lessons. After interpreting and identifying the information, the teacher formulates and implements a lesson plan, which includes strategies that will meet the needs of the individual students and the class as a whole. Implementation may be in the form of large-group instruction, small-group instruction, individualized learning, or peer-to-peer learning.

Each of these delivery strategies serves a specific purpose in the planning of the teacher's lesson. The large-group approach may be used to introduce the lesson and is completed during the readiness phase. This approach captures everyone's attention and begins a process of activating prior knowledge, as well as helping the students see the bigger educational picture.

Once the teacher has identified the objective and Essential Question to the class, then and only then should the Readiness Set activity be completed. In addition, the teacher may find it necessary to link the students' prior knowledge to real-world examples.

A SAMPLE LESSON

The following is an example of a science lesson, developed by Matt Barbiere is an example, comprising all of the components we have discussed in this chapter: As you review the sample lesson plan, please refer back to Figure 1.3 to see the relationships of the various components of the lesson.

Title: Ecology, Habitats, and Food Chains
Lesson: Weird Friends
Essential Question: Why does an ecosystem rely on the living organism's interrelationship within the living and nonliving environmental structure?

Probing Questions

1. What is an ecosystem? (Big picture)
2. How is an ecosystem the same or different from your family? (Compare ecosystem to real-life example)
3. How does a family develop relationships and dependencies between and among family members?

Student Learning Target (Objective)

- I will illustrate the interactions of organisms within an ecosystem, by constructing a Venn diagram and will justify my explanation of relationships of the organisms in the system.
- I will compare and contrast the essential interdependency of an ecosystem and a family. I will be able to compare and contrast the ecosystem and a family and analyze the relationships of the two systems.
- I will be able to create a short story based on the concepts discussed in this lesson using evidence and research to support the facts in the story.
- I will hypothesize about the interconnection between organisms and their environment.

Core Content Curriculum Standards

SCIENTIFIC PROCESSES 5.1: ALL STUDENTS WILL DEVELOP PROBLEM-SOLVING, DECISION-MAKING AND INQUIRY SKILLS, REFLECTED BY FORMULATING USABLE QUESTIONS AND HYPOTHESIS, PLANNING EXPERIMENTS, CONDUCTING SYSTEMATIC OBSERVATIONS, INTERPRETING AND ANALYZING DATA, DRAWING CONCLUSIONS, AND COMMUNICATING SKILLS

Note: Remind students to employ self-regulation strategies throughout the lesson.

- Remind students to use available resources or to *ask a friend for help*, before asking the teacher a question. (Remember students: TBM or Two before Me).
- Remind students to make careful observations of their ecosystems. After the observations, they will record their answers in their journals. They will use the rubrics to self-manage and self-monitor their answers.
- Remind students to keep records that describe observations, to carefully distinguish actual observations from ideas and speculations, and write key concepts. The students will be instructed to manage their time wisely, as note-keeping is a form of self-management, and is an important self-regulation strategy.
- Encourage students to use technology in the classroom (the district may provide laptops or computer carts with student computers or iPods for student use). The goal for the students is to self-manage their learning by seeking out resources.
- Encourage students to actively search for information during their independent time and monitor their progress.
- If the students are going to conduct a science investigation, precise recordkeeping is crucial to the replication of the process of the experiment. During the process, remind students to reflect upon their actions and methods, by continually asking "why" and finally be prepared to justify their activities and answers.
- Encourage students to collaborate and communicate ideas with their peers, as well as to extract information from posters, rubrics, exemplars, or instructional charts, in their surrounding environment. Discuss collaboration and communication as forms of self-regulation and discuss other medium that was used as a form of self-regulation through observation.

LANGUAGE ARTS: 3.2.3 A. WRITING AS A PROCESS (PREWRITING, DRAFTING, REVISING, EDITING, POST-WRITING)

- Generate ideas for writing, through recalling experiences, listening to stories, reading, brainstorming, and discussion.

- Examine real-world examples of writing in various genres, to gain understanding of how authors communicate their ideas through form, structure, and their voice.
- Use graphic organizers to assist with the formal planning while writing.
- Compose first drafts from prewriting work.
- Revise a draft by rereading for meaning, narrowing the focus, sequencing, elaborating with detail, improving openings, closings, and word choice, to show voice.
- Participate with peers to comment on and react to each other's writing.
- Build an awareness of the techniques authors use in their paragraphs to support meaning.
- Begin to develop author's voice in their own writing.
- Use reference materials such as a dictionary, Internet, and other software resources to revise work.

3.2.3 B. WRITING AS A PRODUCT (RESULTING IN A FORMAL PRODUCT OR PUBLICATION)

- Write a descriptive piece, such as a description of a person, place, or object.
- Present and discuss writing with other students.
- Apply elements of grade-appropriate rubrics to improve writing.

3.2.3 C. MECHANICS, SPELLING, HANDWRITING

- Use standard English conventions, which are developmentally appropriate to the grade level, such as sentences, punctuation, capitalization, and spelling.
- Use grade-appropriate knowledge of English grammar and usage, to craft writing, such as singular and plural nouns, subject/verb agreement, and appropriate parts of speech.

3.2.3 D. WRITING FORMS, AUDIENCES, AND PURPOSES (EXPLORING A VARIETY OF FORMS)

- Write for a variety of purposes (e.g., to inform, entertain, persuade) and audiences (e.g., self, peers, community).
- Develop fluency by writing daily and for sustained amounts of time.
- Write the events of a story sequentially.
- Produce writing that demonstrates the use of a variety of sentence types, such as declarative, interrogative, exclamatory, and imperative.

3.3.3 A. DISCUSSION (SMALL GROUP AND WHOLE CLASS)

- Listen and follow a discussion, in order to contribute to the topic appropriately.
- Stay focused on the topic.
- Take turns. (Identify roles for the students, and have the students rotate their roles throughout the lesson.)
- Support an opinion with detail and evidence.

3.3.3 C. WORD CHOICE

- Use vocabulary related to a particular topic.
- Use words from the word wall.

READINESS SET

The teacher will ask the class: What is your favorite sandwich to eat? Ask the students why it is their favorite. Eventually someone will say a peanut butter and jelly sandwich. They seem to go well together, don't they? Can you suggest other examples of two items that work well together? (Ask this question if the students provide sandwiches which are not two selections.)

After an initial discussion about two items that go together, such as peanut butter and jelly, begin a second discussion regarding the new thoughts from students. This new discussion probes what happens if the two selections are not connected.

What would happen if you couldn't make the sandwich by yourself; what would you do? Would you ask for help? Did you receive any help from an unexpected source?

Today we are going to talk about two points: The first point is how things are related and go together in the environment, and the second is about receiving help from an external source.

Let's think about the two questions: first thought, things that go together; and second thought, receiving help. After you reflect upon these two separate thoughts, write a journal entry about your insights and understanding of each of the points. You will have three to four minutes to do this activity, and then we will share our thoughts and writings.

As students share their stories, they will comment on their peers' perceptions and/or discuss these answers in small groups. The students are instructed to take notes on the "relationships" enumerated from the discussions when they began their project.

Students will also learn that there will be time for them to work independently on their project. The independent time will be approximately twenty minutes after the lesson is introduced. This concept of *spacing the lesson* is consistent with "prime time and down time," which is discussed in cognitive research and the learning brain. Specifically, after a certain period of time, there should be a "cooling down" session or "downtime" session when information can be processed.

After this independent time, students will share their class work. Prior to sharing this information, the teacher will remind students about the previous stories which were read in class that were about relationships.

INSTRUCTIONAL INPUT

For this lesson, the teacher will introduce the scholars to the food chain, and the relationship between predators and prey, in the ecosystem, through large group instruction. The class will gain a simple understanding of the ecosystem and its living organisms. The scholars will be given time, during the lesson to work independently or in small groups.

To introduce the idea of animals relying upon each other in the ecosystem, the teacher will read the book *Weird Friends, Unlikely Allies in the Animal Kingdom*. The purpose or objective of this lesson is to inspire the students to think about their family members and how interdependency is created within their own household.

After the book introduction activity, which was reflected on in a large-group setting, the teacher will establish smaller groups of four persons. The teacher will ask each student to identify one animal from the story, and cite examples regarding the animal's relationship with other animals. For example, the teacher may state, "Students, I want you to think about one animal from the story we just read, and then I want you to think about how this animal helped another animal in the story."

A four-square template activity will be facilitated by directing the students to fold a piece of construction paper in half (sometimes called a "hamburger fold") and then in half again, thereby creating four squares. The squares will be numbered one, two, three, and four. The numbering of the squares is important and can be used for a variety of activities.

For example, the teacher may ask students to draw or write down one conflict depicted in a chapter book in square one, and how the conflict was resolved in square two. This visually displays the relationship between the problem and the solution and organizes it in sequential order of one and two, for the student. The students may share what they draw or write with their classmates. Or, children can be grouped according to what they put into the number one square. Students will have the opportunity to explain and justify their reasoning for what they put in each of the squares, as it relates to the chapter book, teachers directions, and their perceptions.

MODELING

During the student small group time, the teacher will share, with the class, a time he or she has received help from an unlikely source. The purpose of sharing the experience is to help the students understand that sometimes you may receive help without asking for help.

INPUT (ACTIVITIES)

The class will sit on the floor and listen to the teacher reading the book. The children will be asked to discuss some of the ideas that were mentioned in the book (pair–share activity).

The students will write a short story about animals helping each other in a given situation. The stories will need to have factual evidence, so students will be asked to use the reference materials (computer, dictionary, books, etc.) in the classroom, to assist with the writing process.

The students will use the four-square templates to organize their ideas and structure of the stories. After they have their ideas set up, the students will write a draft of their story. Next, the student will share the template ideas with a friend. The next step is for the teacher to review the draft with the students and revise, rewrite, and reflect upon the mechanics of their story.

After the review, the students will be asked to write a final copy of their paper. To modify the activity for students who cannot write a story, as stated in their Individualized Education Plans (IEPs), drawing or symbolism will be substituted and the child will be able to dictate his or her thoughts orally to the teacher or assistant. These picture stories will be done the same way as the written ones. They will need to use a four-square template, "draft copy," and make their good copies for the stories.

CHECK FOR UNDERSTANDING

During the activity, there will be frequent checks for understanding using a variety of strategies. The teacher will need to periodically determine if the children understand what was being taught. Their answers will be shared with the class. During that time, the students will be chosen randomly by each other. Each student will have an opportunity to call upon other students (popcorn activity), creating a cycle of involvement and discussion where everyone is engaged for a common reason.

The calling on students will ensure that all children are participating. Participation is not an option. At this time, the class will construct a KWL (also known as KWHL chart: what you *K*now, what you *W*ant to know *H*ow you learned it, and what you *L*earned) chart based upon the answer sheets.

This chart will show what the class already knows, learned, how they got their answers, and what they want to learn from the lesson. This chart will be posted at the top of the classroom and will supplement continually as new information is learned and/or needed to be learned. This chart should serve as a resource and be available throughout the lesson.

USING MULTIPLE INTELLIGENCES

Linguistic: The students will be asked to write a short story about a time when they may have relied on someone or something. During the writing experience time, the students will brainstorm first. To help organize their stories, they will construct a four-square writing template and sequence it starting from square one to square four.

Students will be asked to write a draft of their short stories. While the students write these stories, they will be reminded to refer to the writing rubrics and writing exemplars, so they can begin the process of self-correcting and self-monitoring. The draft will be reviewed by the teacher and the students together to show the students' possible mistakes, but most importantly, to discuss the students' strengths and weaknesses in composition.

During the activity, feedback is important for improvement as it provides correction and encouragement. These stories will be expected to have factual evidence in them, and will be asked to *not* be completely fiction. The students will be expected to use facts that they discovered during the lesson. They can also use the reference materials available in the classroom for further assistance.

Logical–Mathematical

The students will create a board game showing interrelationships.

Musical

Have the children attempt a rhyming poem or metaphor in order to bring life and a personal understanding of the animals and their environment. For example; The lion was "ty-in" . . . his shoelaces! The children might also construct a rhyming book. In order to create fluidness in rhythm, the children will add a drumbeat when chanting "lion" and "ty-in" to keep the book flowing smoothly. This is a great way to influence learning.

Bodily Kinesthetic

The students will write/create a play and act it out.

Spatial–Visual

The children create a graphic representation of a concept, idea, or process.

Interpersonal

After a discussion with the class, about the friendships described in *Frog and Toad Are Friends*, a first grade reader (or continue with the book named above, *Weird Friends, Unlikely Allies in the Animal Kingdom*), the teacher will ask students, "Which friendship was most interesting to you?"

The student will be asked to turn to the page of the friendship book that the student shared with the class, and have the student lead a discussion about the interdependency of the animals. Have the students give examples of friendships they made in and out of school. Make time to do this with several different animal partnerships described in the book.

Intrapersonal

Read the book *Weird Friends Unlikely Allies in the Animal Kingdom* to the class. The book discusses the dependency of diverse animals upon each other, which ultimately aids in their worldly survival. Have a discussion among the students about the relationships that they discovered during the reading. Have the students discuss them in class. Use visualization; have students close their eyes to think about and picture relationships.

Naturalist

Have the students construct and describe an ecosystem in nature.

Accommodations

The students will be asked to listen to the book and answer questions, through pictures, which support relationships. The students may also use manipulatives to show relationships. The students will also be able to visually represent relationships through drawings or by acting out the relationships.

Guided Practice and Monitoring

During the student's guided practice time, the teacher will walk around the room and monitor the students' work. The teacher will use the strategy "Praise, Prompt, Leave." (This author requests that you make the praise fulfilling and not empty praise, which is discussed in later in chapter.)

When the students complete their work, they will meet with the teacher to review their draft and make necessary corrections. After this conference, the students will write a final draft. As the students complete their final copies, they will be asked to assist with the correcting of the papers of other students who need extra help.

Assessments

Various assessments will be applied during the learning process as detailed assessments are denoted in chapter 2.

Consolidation for Closure

The teacher will say: "Since we discussed in class the idea of teamwork in the ecosystem and how they help manage the balance represented in the ecosystem, tell your neighbor one thing you learned today" (covert closure). After you pair–share, be prepared to report out what you heard.

As another example of the closure, the student will create a "3–2–1 card." On an index card, the students will write three things they learned, two things they were confused about, and one thing stating how they came to their conclusions.

Since the inclusion of "*H*" for "*H*ow they did it," the author suggests renaming 3–2–1 to 3–2–1 Blamed. At a blastoff signal (clap of the teacher's hand), the student shares with his or her peers and the teacher *H*ow the sequence of events leads to learning.

Independent Practice

Have the students go home and examine the interactions in their own houses. Ask the children to write about what would happen if one person did not do his or her job at home.

As noted earlier and shown in the graphic later, the informational stage involves providing teacher-directed instruction, student-directed instruction, independent work, small-group activities, and/or cooperative activities. All of these strategies are part of the instructional delivery. Please refer to Figure 1.1 in Chapter 1 for a schema of this delivery.

The delivery phase begins with a teacher-directed instruction (large-group instruction) Please refer to Figure 1.2 for a schema. During the course of the instructional delivery phase, there are techniques that can be employed which will enhance student achievement. These techniques can be verbal (linguistic) or nonlinguistic.

Nonlinguistic representations can include the use of mental imagery. For example, think about X. Can you see X in your mind's eye? Or have students draw a representation or make a graphic or visual organizer. The graphic or visual organizer can take on many forms.

A concept map is one example of an organizer. The map would be useful in organizing and representing the relationships in a variety of ways. For example, the concept map can look like a spider, with the main concept in the center and auxiliary branches protruding from the center.

An organizational chart in the form of a chain is another type of concept map. Be mindful when deciding upon a map, because each form has characteristics and advantages over the other forms and your choice of organizer is hinged upon your objectives and goals for learning. If one wants to illustrate a concept showing the relationships with similarities and differences, then a "spider model" would be useful. A spider diagram will have a body with lines coming off the body and nodes coming off the lines.

To define relationships by showing subordinates or superordinates, the hierarchy chart would be a better choice. Using a school district, as an example of a hierarchy map, one would list the Board of Education at the top,

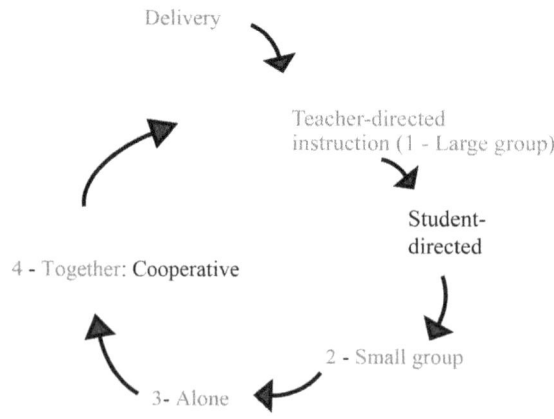

Figure 1.2

with the superintendent reporting to the Board of Education. Below the superintendent would be the business administrator and assistant superintendents, followed by directors, principals, vice principals, supervisors, coordinators, teachers, and staff.

To develop a time line of sequence, a chain map would be used with the tasks defined, objectives, benchmarks, and activities identified. Many teachers have used story maps (title, main idea, supporting information) or analogy maps, which show new and familiar concepts.

SMALL-GROUP ACTIVITY AND COOPERATIVE LEARNING STRATEGIES SUGGESTIONS

When working in small groups or using cooperative learning activities, the following are a few suggestions:

- Organizing groups can be based on ability level or organized into groups by varied skill levels.
- Cooperative groups should be kept small so the teacher can monitor the group to assess student progress and so individuals in the group can participate.
- Cooperative learning should be constructed for a purpose not to have an activity where students are doing a project or activity in groups. It is ineffective when it is not purposeful, planned, and guided. An activity that is not planned is not a purposeful activity; an activity that is planned is a purposeful activity because it will lead to something.
- Small cooperative groups are more effective when the activity is planned and all students have the opportunity to participate. Group members have specific roles; there are protocols for everyone having a "voice" and an expected outcome.
- Cooperative groups should be monitored as there is a tendency for one person to control the group. With a strong personality in the group, students may defer to a strong personality or not even contribute.

As mentioned earlier, practice is important. However, practice should be rendered so that it reinforces those skills expected to be learned. Teachers need to be mindful about practice.

THE CONCEPT OF PRACTICE

Practice will make perfect, so when repeating the same thing over and over, one engages in practice. The critical point is that the practice must be perfect practice. Perfect practice, such as writing the multiplication tables correctly, will make the practice "perfect" learning.

Conditions to Consider for Practice

- The learner, who engages in practice, must be focused on self-management with the understanding that practice will lead to improved performance. A baseball player engages in batting practices so when he is in a game his performance will increase.
- During the practice, the student should engage in self-regulated learning (SRL).
- Prior to engaging in practice, the learner must know exactly what is to be practiced. If it is a skill to be learned for procedural knowledge, like learning the multiplication tables, then repetition is useful as the skill is learned so it becomes second nature.
- If a concept is to be learned, the learner must know what the concept is as there may be multiple ways to solve the problem and if it is an application problem, the learner must have the necessary skills for the application to be solved.
- In order to create something, the learner must have the competency skills to perform. If you seek performance you need competency; if you seek competency, you may not get performance.
- The learner should reflect after the activity so he or she can self-regulate his or her learning in subsequent activities.
- The learner should seek feedback from the homework so the feedback can be used for self-managing future tasks. The process can involve journaling or conferencing with the teacher.
- Once feedback is given, the learner will know how to modify or adapt his or her learning.

As a teacher, it is important that the grouping process begins correctly for the student. The adage "Well begun is half done" is relevant. The teacher should plan for the grouping model to ensure the groups are proceeding correctly. Once the teacher feels comfortable with what the student is doing, then the students can progress.

After the teacher feels comfortable with the progress of the lesson, keeping in mind the notion of primacy-recency, there may be a point in the lesson for students to do independent practice. The teacher needs to monitor the student's progress and ensure that the student has the knowledge and appropriate skill to do the activity independently.

Marzano, Pickering, and Pollock produced a chart in their book *Classroom Instruction That Works: Research Based Strategies for Increasing Student*

Lesson Delivery 21

Guided practice cycle – alone (as determined by the pace of the lesson)

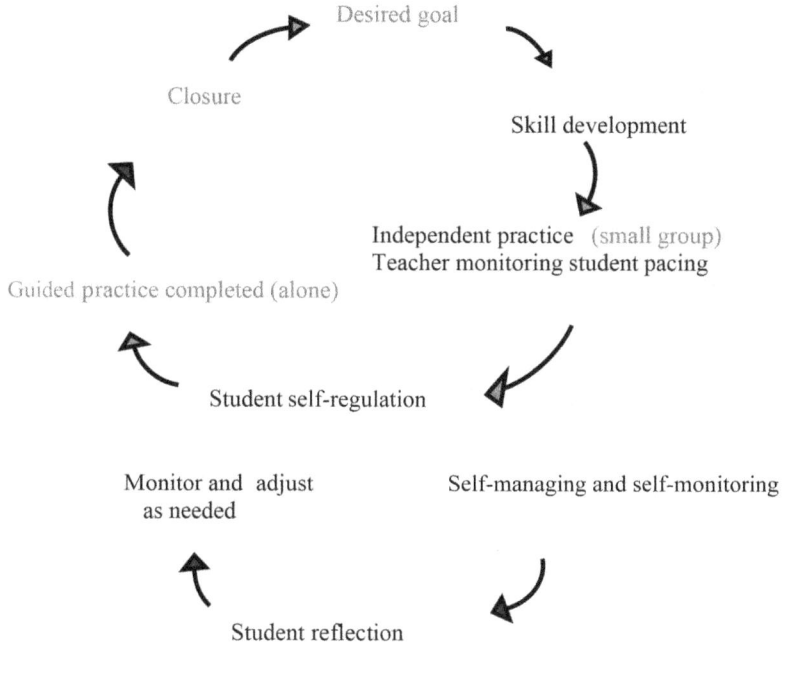

Guided practice (individual)

Figure 1.3

Achievement in which the cumulative percentage increase for the first four practice sessions will yield a 47.9 percent increase. Four additional practice sessions yield only an additional 14 percent additional increase (from 47.9 to 61.2 percent).

Eight practice sessions yield a total of 61.2 percent gain. Six additional practice sessions, for a total of sixteen practice sessions, will result in an increase to 71.4 percent. The eight additional practice sessions for a total of twenty-four sessions will yield the 80.4 percent gain (Marzano, Pickering, and Pollock 2001, 68).

Not only must the student be guided to ensure that he or she is beginning the assignment knowing what to do, but he or she must also practice the assignments over and over again, for an increase in achievement to occur. As noted earlier, the more perfect the practice, the better the results.

Normally, home learning is the chosen form of practice. Many educators believe in the academic and nonacademic benefits of home learning for all grade and ability levels, which is why it serves as an impetus for continued educational practice. It is also acknowledged as a valuable part of the learning process. However, home learning can be busywork for students that will have limited or no value at all so teachers must be mindful in developing homework assignments so the assignment is purposeful and deliberate. What are the types of practice a student can use?

MASSED PRACTICE OR DISTRIBUTED PRACTICE

Massed Practice

Research suggests a pattern of practice that is twofold, massed practice and distributed practice. Massed practice is practicing a new learning during time periods that are very close together. Sustained practice over time is called "distributed practice." Each pattern has an advantage and is used in different scenarios. Any college student who studied for a test the night before the test engaged in "massed practice." In reality, massed practice is effective because the brain consolidates information from the day during the night.

When studying of information at night, the information that was studied gets stored while you sleep, the next day walking into a classroom to take a test after cramming all night for a test, the student feels "don't bump into me, or else everything will fall out of my brain." The downside to massed practice is the information usually does not go into long-term memory and is quickly forgotten. It is not uncommon for the information to be forgotten after a few days.

Distributed Practice

To develop long-term memory, a better practice to use is called "distributed practice." Distributed practice involves spacing the practice or studying over a period of time. A student may study for a test two months before the test, then restudy four weeks before the exam, then review two days before the exam. In this model, the studying is spaced out over a period of time.

This concept of distributed practice corresponds to the research by Marzano, Pickering, and Pollock (2001), in which the initial growth will occur over a period of time (47 percent increase after four practice sessions and 61 percent increase after ten practice activities). For the greater gain of 80 percent, it will require fourteen more sessions.

An example of the two types of practice is when we try to remember a telephone number. When we want to remember a person's phone number, we may write it down a few times, so we can memorize it. After repeated practice, we will eventually remember the number. The number has been "massed practiced," and then "distributed practiced."

More importantly, the number has meaning and makes sense because that person or situation associated with the number is important to us, at least for the moment. Sense and meaning will help commit the number to memory.

The following are some suggestions for pre-home learning questions whether the student is practicing massed or distributed practice.

- Tell the class the Essential Question they will be working on in the future.
- Provide a list of keywords that will be covered in the next unit.
- Ask the class to think about what they learned and what they will be studying.
- Have students make a Venn diagram to show the relationships.
- Create a real-world scenario or physical representation.
- Promote self-regulation strategies of student self-management by having the students find facts about the new topic.

INDEPENDENT PRACTICE

Regarding independent practice (which should begin in school and continue at home), a critical practice for success is when the teacher checks for student understanding throughout the lesson, and adjusts the lesson according to the needs of the students. This phase is important so the teacher will know if the student is ready to do the task during independent practice.

The check for understanding involves having the teacher elicit responses from students, for the purpose of gathering information, as to whether or not they comprehend the skills or if there is a need to make an immediate adjustment in the lesson. There are common pitfalls when checking for understanding, which should be avoided.

Checking for Understanding Pitfalls

- The most common mistake a teacher makes is asking the class if everyone is "OK." The problem is that few, if any, students will say that they are confused or not "OK" because it will appear that they are "stupid."
- The assumption that everything is OK because the students are silent is incorrect reasoning on the teacher's part.
- Another common (and also ineffective) way to check student understanding is a statement by the teacher that everyone understands what was taught: "You all have it, right?" Here again students will be reluctant to report that they do not understand the material.

- Another ineffective method for checking student understanding is the query "Now does anyone have a question?" The implication is that if you have a question about the material you are not as smart as the students who do not have questions.

Keeping these common errors in mind, how does a teacher check for understanding so that changes to the instructional delivery may be made to build success within individuals and within the classroom environment? Suggestions include sampling students to see if a variety of students comprehend the material, using signaling, having students provide feedback via whiteboards, or using response clickers or other vehicles that gather individual information.

Each practice is used to provide feedback to the teacher. Sampling would involve calling on a random sample of students in the class to share an answer. Based on the feedback received, the teacher will make an informal assessment of how the lesson is progressing.

In a study of twenty-six high-achieving, high-poverty schools in Texas, researchers identified teachers' ability to accurately identify student needs, through the use of assessments and other "reflection" tools, and to plan instruction accordingly, as a common characteristic of successful classrooms (Johnson 1998). The researchers found that the use of formative assessments enabled the teacher to assess the students in the class and determine how students are progressing through the lesson.

The assessments allowed teachers to determine the strengths, weaknesses, and progress of the students which was useful information for the teacher who can then help the students use self-regulation strategies for their individual growth. After the assessments are made, the teacher can modify the student's learning environment to facilitate the self-regulation process.

Specific Strategies to Use

Some specific strategies that can be incorporated into any lesson during any instructional phase of the Learner's Brain Model include:

- To help students consolidate their learning and develop sense and meaning from the lesson, have students summarize their learning. Typically this is done as a consolidation for closure activity, but it can also be a home learning task.
- Have students identify similarities and differences.
- Throughout the lesson, have students understand the critical attributes of what they are learning and have them identify similarities and differences between and among concepts. Venn diagrams and T-charts are useful for this activity.

Lesson Delivery 25

- Use metaphors and analogies.
- Stories are powerful memory tools as well as metaphors and analogies. Be mindful that the stories are relevant to what is being taught and not a "walk down memory lane" or "a war story."
- Present material nonlinguistically.
- Use visual representations or manipulatives as part of the instructional delivery as every auditory experience requires a visual representation so students are exposed to a multisensory experience.
- Create and test a hypothesis.
- Have students predict what will happen and create and test hypothesis.
- Reinforce effort of positive recognition for the accomplishments. Provide positive recognition for accomplishments. Teachers should be specific in the feedback that is given to students.
- Promote a growth mind-set. Use the word "yet" to help students that they have not reached the correct answer yet but with a little help they will get it.
- Assign home learning and provide practice. Reinforce lessons with practice and/or home learning.
- Facilitate and monitor cooperative learning.
- Have students work in pairs or groups and share their thinking.
- Set objectives and provide feedback throughout the cooperative lesson.
- Begin the process of self-regulation by setting student learning targets for each group in the cooperative arrangement.
- Provide feedback to students throughout the cooperative lesson so they can self-regulate their learning.
- Start and reinforce activities with clues, questions, and advance organizers.
- Use Readiness Set to begin the lesson and follow up with clues, questions, and multiple representations throughout the lesson, and close with a consolidation closer.

If we rearrange the list in another way, the order may be even more advantageous:

- Begin the process of self-regulation by setting student learning targets and providing feedback to students throughout the lesson so they can self-regulate their learning.
- Posting objectives begins the process of self-regulation on the students' part. Encourage and promote student self-regulation.
- Most importantly, it is necessary for the teacher to use prompts or gestures to refer back to the objective(s) and the Essential Question, in order to focus student attention and "forward frame" the information for future use.

Use a Readiness Set to begin the lesson and follow up with clues, questions, and multiple representations throughout the lesson, and close with a consolidation closer.

- As research indicates, there would be gains when student readiness is promoted.
- Research on lesson design promotes student readiness by starting a lesson using a Readiness Set.
- The Readiness Set helps to bridge prior knowledge, with new information to motivate, as well as focus the student's attention.

Have students predict what will happen and create and test a hypothesis.

- If the students are exposed to a Readiness Set, then as the lesson begins, ask them to predict/ hypothesize what will happen next. This will be useful for students who are beginning the inquiry process.
- Encourage students to "dig deeper," by using critical-thinking skills to learn the subject matter.
- Encourage students to see the horizontal relationship between disparate pieces of information (horizontal articulation) and encourage them to understand how the information is connected and tied to the big picture (vertical articulation).

Present material using a variety of modalities, not just linguistically. Use visual representations or manipulatives as part of the instructional delivery.

- This is an important concept, as it allows for more than one modality to be explored and used in presentation.
- For tactile learners, teachers may choose graphic organizers, study charts, and multiple intelligence strategies, which all involve different types of instructional delivery, while addressing individual learning styles.
- For the auditory learners, teachers can have students work in groups or with a partners to discuss and explain what they are learning. Talking about concepts is beneficial, as it enhances the visual and nonlinguistic representations students construct.

Throughout the lesson:

- Have students understand the critical attributes of what they are learning and identify similarities and differences between and among concepts.
- Use multiple representations like Venn diagram, which is an excellent strategy for students as they discriminate between "what is the same and what is

different." More importantly, the process promotes the higher-level thinking of analysis, synthesis, and evaluation.
- Have students analyze concepts and develop a rationale.
- Uses metaphors and analogies. Stories are powerful memory tools as well as metaphors and analogies. Be mindful that the stories are relevant to what is being taught. More importantly the story will be remembered, so make sure it is germane to a main point.

STORIES AND ANALOGIES

As stated earlier, stories are psychologically privileged when they are stored in the brain. A story has the information stored as an entity and consequently retrieved in its entirety, as opposed to having information stored in various parts of the brain, and the retrieval process involves pulling information from the various sections.

ANALOGIES

Additionally, using metaphors and analogies will be very useful to engage the students in higher-order thinking skills. Who among us can forget the experiences we had when either doing analogies or taking the Miller Analogy Test? Teaching analogy lessons on the chalkboard or doing a classroom assessment helps one to observe how and why our students select key relationships, between the two facts, resulting in the creation of that perfect analogy.

Ideas for extending the analogy can include asking students to explain the relationship, work in pairs to expand it, critique or generate additional analogies, or use the analogies as a study guide for further research.

Keep in mind that using analogies can be very difficult for some students, which may be frustrating and cause them to shut down. Therefore, it may be necessary for a teacher to monitor the instruction. Do frequent checks for understanding, observe genuine engagement among students, ensure all students understand the concept, and all students are able to complete one analogy with a partner, proving they fully understand the concepts being taught.

REINFORCE EFFORT

Reinforce effort and provide positive recognition for accomplishments. Promote a growth mind-set and provide positive recognition for accomplishments. Be specific in the feedback that is given to students.

There is a difference between belief and effort. If the student believes he or she has the ability to score high on a test, he or she will do well. This same student may believe he or she lacks the necessary skills to complete the test; therefore, he or she may not even attempt the test at all. Students who do not feel they have the ability to do a specific task ultimately will not achieve.

The key to success is that the teacher promotes a growth mind-set to drive students to a higher level. If students believe that effort is most important factor in achievement, it will motivate them to try in any situation. If a student perceives they have a high level of ability, but it is shadowed by fear, the student may not do well on a test. This will cause them to think something is wrong and question their belief in their ability.

Effort, on the other hand, can be taught and linked to achievement. Effective teachers say: "I know you can do this, let's try little harder and next time I know you will do better." Praise that explicitly acknowledges the connection between the students' additional effort and their specific achievement, rather than praise for intelligence, causes them to work more, experience more enjoyment, and be more persistent in tasks. There are numerous biographies, autobiographies, and/or stories that serve as examples of how human effort resulted in achievement.

STRATEGIES TO PROMOTE METACOGNITION

Facilitate cooperative learning. Have students work in pairs or groups and share their thinking. It is the environment of cooperative learning that supports that students are afforded the opportunity to share and discuss ideas, as well as engage in metacognition.

PROMOTE ENGAGEMENT

One example at the elementary level is when a teacher assigned a number from one to twelve to her students. After the lesson was presented, the teacher asked all the students who had "ones" to meet together and all the "twos" to meet together and so on. The teacher also arranged for different configurations, by having ones and threes or the ones and fours meet.

The social dynamics that were created by this exercise are fascinating, and much is learned through collaborative and cooperative education. Leaders, followers, stressors, and more points are identified when groups are formed.

Ask students to write a summary of the lesson. To help students consolidate their learning and develop sense and meaning from the lesson, have students summarize their learning. Typically this is done as a consolidation for closure activity but it can also be a home learning task. This activity could be considered either a formative assessment or a closure activity.

If the activity is used as a closure activity, it is important that the teachers use the information that was gathered by them or by the class. If the teachers want to use a formative assessment, then they could use the "Muddiest Point."

This strategy depicts something the student is not clear about which can be used as a check for understanding or a formative assessment. A variation of this assessment would be a "cloudy point" where something is not clear to the student and is noted on an index card.

The "critical point" is the point where students begin to self-regulate their own learning, as they are reviewing the lesson material and assessing important documentation, and they determine if further explanations are required (muddy point). Finally, the student will decide what they need to do to clarify any confusion. At this point, students are now engaged in their learning and can decipher what is important and what needs clarity in order to complete their task.

PROMOTE HOME LEARNING

Assign home learning to provide practice. Reinforce lessons with practice and/or home learning. Home learning, by itself, is not the solution to ensure that students will understand and apply the skills which were taught.

The following are the basic generalizations about home learning:

- The amount of home learning assigned to students should be different for elementary, middle school, and high school students.
- Most districts have policies on how much home learning can be assigned to students, so be mindful of district policy.
- Home learning is to reinforce a skill or a concept so it has a meaning.
- Parental involvement in home learning should be kept to a minimum.
- The purpose of home learning should be identified and articulated so the student will know what to do when they get home.
- Home learning is for the student and not the parent.
- The parent sets the environment and checks on the student to ensure that the work is getting done.
- If home learning is assigned, it should be commented on by the teacher as teacher feedback is very important for student self-regulation.

RESEARCH ON HOME LEARNING

Cooper, Robinson, and Patall (2006) conducted a meta-analysis of the research in the United States between 1987 and 2003 that examined home learning effectiveness. The researchers identified four instructional purposes of homework: (1) to practice or review content already covered in class, (2) to become acquainted with new material that will be covered in a subsequent class, (3) to extend understanding of previously learned content to new situations, and (4) to integrate separate content and skills. Through this meta-analysis it was concluded that a positive relationship exists between homework and student achievement, though no distinction was made between pre-homework and traditional practice homework.

What Do the Proponents Say about Home Learning? The practice of newly learned skills strengthens the acquisition of content, thus enhancing overall academic performance. Academically speaking, the benefits of home learning include developing and maintaining scholastic skills through practice with the intent of the student becoming proficient and mastering new material. In addition to skill enhancement, homework promotes nonacademic benefits, including learning how to work independently, developing time-management skills, involving the parents in their child's education, promoting effective study habits, and improving students' attitudes toward school.

Additionally, at the middle and high school level, students may have seven or eight teachers in the course of a day. If every teacher assigned thirty minutes of home learning, it would take several hours to complete all the assignments. District should have policies and procedures to resolve this problem, especially since it is the quality of homework that counts.

The other consideration regarding home learning is that it should be assigned for a specific purpose and for the student's personal gain and benefit. Parents want to be helpful and do the home learning for the child, but since the parents were not present during class, when the information was provided, it would be difficult to understand how and to what extent one should be helpful.

Finally, another consideration regarding home learning is not how it reinforces skills but how it can help a student do well on a test or quiz. In the next chapter, we will see the most important point regarding home learning: feedback, which is highly valuable for the student. Feedback helps students to self-regulate and to produce achievement. In other words, home learning for the sake of home learning will not yield results. Home learning should not be busy work.

The next chapter provides ways in which home learning and assessments can promote learning.

Please refer to appendix B for a rubric on student engagement that can be used for planning a lesson to assess a lesson. Remember, compliance does not mean engagement.

BIBLIOGRAPHY

Angelo, T. A., and K. P. Cross. 1993. *Classroom Assessment Techniques: A Handbook for College Teachers*, 2nd edition. San Francisco, CA: Jossey-Boss, Inc.

Chipman, S. P., and R. Glaser, eds. *Thinking and Learning Skills: Relating Instruction to Research*, Vol. 1. Hillsdale, NJ: Lawrence Erlbaum, 389–416.

Cooper, H. 1989a. *Homework*. White Plains, NY: Longman Publishing Company.

———. 1989b. "Synthesis of Research on Homework." *Educational Leadership* 47 (30): 85–91.

Cooper, H., Robinson, J. C., and Patall, E. A. 2006. "Does homework improve academic achievement? A synthesis of research, 1987–2003." *Review of Educational Research* 76 (1): 1–62.

Covington, M. V. 1983. "Motivation Cognitions." In *Learning and Motivation in the Classroom*, ed. S. G. Paris, G. M. Olson, and W. Stevenson, 139–164. Hillsdale, NJ: Laurence Erlbaum.

———. 1985. "Strategic Thinking and the Fear of Failure." In *Thinking and Learning Skills: Relating Instruction to Research*, Vol. 1, ed. J. W. Segal, S. P. Chipman, and R. Glaser, 389–416. Hillsdale, NJ: Erlbaum.

Craske, M. L. 1985. "Improving Persistence through Observational Learning and Attribution Retraining." *British Journal of Educational Psychology* 55: 138–47.

Ebbinghaus, H. 1885. *Memory: A Contribution to Experimental Psychology*. Translated by Henry A. Ruger and Clare E. Bussenius, 1913 edition. New York: Teachers College.

Hermann, D. J., H. Weingartnerm, A. Searleman, and C. McEvoy. 1992. *Memory Improvement: Implications for Memory*. New York: Springer-Verlag.

Hunter, M. 1979, October. "Teaching Is Decision Making." *Educational Leadership* 37 (1): 62–67.

———. 1982. *Mastery Teaching*. El Segundo, CA: TIP Publications.

Jensen, E. 2010. *Different Brains, Different Learners: How to Reach the Hard to Reach*. Thousand Oaks, CA: Corwin Press.

Johnson, B. 1998. The relationships between elementary teachers' perceptions of school climate, student achievement, teacher characteristics, and community and school context (Doctoral dissertation, University of New Mexico, 1998). *Dissertation Abstracts International*, 59 (11), 4055.

Jones, Karrie A., Paul J. Vermette, and Jennifer L. Jones. Winter 2009. "An Integration of 'Backwards Planning' Unit Design with the 'Two-Step' Lesson Planning Framework." *Education* 130 (2): 357–60.

Lynch, Ann Marie, Lea A. Theodore, Melissa A. Bray, and Thomas J. Kehle. 2009. "A Comparison of Group-Oriented Contingencies and Randomized Reinforcers to Improve Homework Completion and Accuracy for Students with Disabilities." *School Psychology Review* 38 (3): 307–24.

Marzano, R. J. 2007. *The Art and Science of Teaching: A Comprehensive Framework for Effective Instruction*. Alexandria, VA: Association for Supervision and Curriculum Development.

Marzano, R. J., D. Pickering, and Jane E. Pollock. 2001. *Classroom Instruction That Works: Research-Based Strategies for Increasing Student Achievement.* Alexandria, VA: Association for Supervision and Curriculum Development.

Mireles, Selina Vásquez, Theresa Westbrook, Debra D. Ward, Joshua Goodson, and Jae Hak Jung. Spring 2013. "Implementing Pre-Homework in the Developmental Mathematics Classroom." *Research & Teaching in Developmental Education* 29 (2): 1–9.

Mueller, C. M., and C. S. Dweck. 1998. "Intelligence Praise Can Undermine Motivation and Performance." *Journal of Personality and Social Psychology* 75 (1): 33–52.

Nadel, Sybil G. 2003. *Instructional Theory into Practice: Instructional Skills.* Trenton: New Jersey Department of Education, Academy for the Advancement of Teaching and Management.

Sousa, D. A. 2001. *How the Special Needs Brain Learns.* Thousand Oaks, CA: Corwin Press.

Stiggins, R. 2005a. "From Formative Assessment to Assessment FOR Learning: A Path to Success in Standards-Based Schools." *Phi Delta Kappan* 86: 324–28.

———. 2005b. *Student-Involved Assessment FOR Learning*, 4th edition. Upper Saddle River, NJ: Pearson Education.

Stiggins, R., and J. Chappuis. 2005. "Using Student-Involved Classroom Assessment to Close Achievement Gaps." *Theory into Practice* 44: 11–18.

Tomlinson, C., and J. McTighe. 2006. *Integrating Differentiation and Understanding by Design: Connecting Content and Kids.* Alexandria, VA: Association for Supervision and Curriculum Development.

Willis, J. 2006. *Research-Based Strategies to Ignite Student Learning: Insights from a Neurologist and Classroom Teacher.* Alexandria, VA: Association for Supervision and Curriculum Development.

Wilson, T. D., and P. W. Linville. 1982. "Improving the Academic Performance of College Freshmen: Attribution Theory Revisited." *Journal of Personal and Social Psychology* 42: 367–76.

Chapter 2

Using Assessments

FOCUS OF THE CHAPTER

Using assessments not for a summative evaluation of learning but for formative assessment of learning to drive instructional practice and delivery is the focus of the chapter. The task is not to just collect data ("data rich") but to analyze what was collected so it can be applied to improve instruction. The lack of not analyzing the data will lead to the adage: "data rich and analysis poor."

INTRODUCTION

As you read this chapter, pleaes keep in mind the following three questions: Is testing the students or teachers friend or foe? How can assessments be used for learning and not of learning? Do assessments deteremine the effectiveness of a lesson?

Probing Questions

1. Are assessments for learning or of learning?
2. Masses or distributed learning?
3. How do I know if students are learning throughout the lesson?
4. How can I use visual, auditory, kinesthetic, or tactile checks of understanding to assess student learning?

ARE ASSESSMENTS THE TEACHER'S FRIEND OR FOE?

Tests and assessments can be a teacher or a student's friends or foe. They can be a student's foe if a student takes a test, does poorly, and becomes discouraged frustrated or upset. However, tests and assessments can be a friend if the student uses a study test protocol instead of a study process. For a study process, the student reads or re-reads his or her notes to become familiar with the information. In a study test protocol, the student studies the material for a period of time, then tests himself or herself to see what he or she recalls.

In the study test protocol, the student is using tests (or assessments) to guide him or her in the learning process. After the initial assessment, the student can reflect on what he or she answered correctly and what needs to be studied. Too often students will review material and become "familiar" with it but may not be able to interpret or explain it. Have you heard students say: "Oh, that looks familiar."

ASKING WHY QUESTIONS

To further enhance the learning process, the student can ask himself or herself the why questions. Why does that matter? Why is that important? Why did they do X? The why questions are meant to develop a better understanding of the material being read and/or help make meaning for the student. The read-pause-reflect cycle will help promote metacognition for the student. (See Roediger and Pye [2012], for research on this practice.)

USING ASSESSMENTS AS AN INSTRUCTIONAL STRATEGY

The teacher can use assessments prior to the test for monitoring and adjusting the students' learning; the assessment strategies are done throughout the instructional period to determine if the students know or understand the material, thereby enabling the teacher to pace his or her lesson.

Additionally, tests can be used for improvement of learning or as a way for students to study. In the former case, assessments are done during the instructions by the teacher, and in the latter, strategies are done during the time set aside for home learning by the student to help improve his or her learning via self-regulation. If the goal is to develop self-regulated learners, it is the student who must engage in the assessment to promote self-regulation, self-monitoring, or self-management

The question becomes, how can teachers employ various strategies to help promote student learning and student self-regulation by using assessments or tests? An additional question is, how can students use their assessments to enhance their learning?

STUDENT USE OF ASSESSMENTS FOR SELF-REGULATION

The conventional thinking of assessments is that teachers provide instructional information and an assessment is given so the teachers can determine if the instruction was effective (summative evaluation). This protocol directs the process of learning from the teacher to student. How can the teacher help the student to direct or assess his or her own learning and promote the use of test and assessments for the self-regulation process?

If the students were to engage in a teacher-directed protocol, the teacher must develop a feedback loop emanating from the student back to the teacher. The critical component of the loop is the students' use of assessments for the purpose of Self-Regulated Learning (SRL) and gives feedback to the teacher or is able to self-monitor their work. This is an especially important step in self-regulation.

Promoting Self-Regulation: First Step

The first step in the self-regulation loop process would be to ensure that students understand SRL strategies so they can employ strategies when a teacher is not available. In order for this to occur, self-regulating learning strategies must be taught by the teachers and usually the earlier the better. Teachers should model the process whenever possible and explain to students what they are doing so students understand that they are learning a process.

Promoting Self-Regulation: Second Step

The second step for self-regulation is to construct a classroom environment that promotes student self-regulation. The self-regulated classroom provides rubrics, exemplars, meaningful environment, encourages the use of journals, work folders, and portfolios to construct a learning environment students can use for self-regulation.

However, just the construction of the learning environment with rubrics and exemplars will not promote self-regulation as the students may soon ignore the information as it becomes blended into the room and loses its meaning and effectiveness; the teacher must tell the students that it is their responsibility to promote their own learning through self-regulation and using the learning environment in the process. Therefore, the teacher reminds the students that they have responsibility for their own learning.

Promoting Self-Regulation: Third Step

The teacher may tell the class: "I want to remind you that throughout the lesson I will be monitoring your progress and I may also want you to monitor your own progress. I will provide self-regulation strategies throughout the lesson; however, I ask that you monitor your progress in one of the two ways:

1. Use the rubrics and exemplars which are posted throughout the room to assess how you are doing. Feel free to get up out of your desk to use the resources in the room.
2. Tonight while you are doing your home learning, continue to use assessments to gauge your learning."

Promoting Students to Self-Regulate: TBM

The teaching of self-regulation concepts is necessary as some students are more inclined to self-regulate their learning than others so all students must be aware of the process and know what to do. As the teacher teaches the lesson, students are reminded that if they are having difficulties, they are to seek out help in other ways before they come to the teacher.

This process of Two Before Me or Three Before Me (TBM) encourages students to get into the habit of seeking resolutions to their problems. TBM can include students talking to other students, using the Internet for research, using reference charts, or employing strategies that the students have been taught to seek a resolution to the problem. In this protocol, learners are seeking alternative ways to resolve a problem before they go to the teacher.

Self-regulation is an invaluable concept to develop as teachers may not always be available to help students when they are working on their projects. How many times has an administrator seen students lined up by a teacher's desk waiting for his or her feedback on an assignment? The students need to be empowered to take ownership of their learning and not be enabled—be self-dependent and not teacher-dependent.

For students in the lower grades, a rubric can be developed for students to use in the assessment of their own learning. Figure 2.1 is an example of a rubric developed by Christine Castle, teacher in Elizabeth Public Schools. She uses this with her first grade students, and they love the visuals. Since the *Jersey Shore* is a big part of the students' life in New Jersey, it is no surprise the students would love a rubric with fish.

USING ASSESSMENTS AND TESTS FOR LEARNING

How do teachers make lessons successful? How do teachers monitor student progress using formative and summative assessments? How does data drive instruction? These are all questions surrounding assessments and, more

Using Assessments 37

BE A SHARK !!
Open Ended Responses

1	2	3	4
Guppy	Flounder	Piranha	SHARK!!!
Good start... *What is needed to become a shark?*	Keep working hard! *What is needed to become a shark?*	You are almost there! *What is needed to become a shark?*	You are fierce! • Uses RACES
• Does not restate the question	• May not restate the question	• Restates the question	• Clearly **R**estates the question
• May not answer all parts/or may not answer completely	• **A**nswers all parts	• **A**nswers all parts	• **A**nswers all parts of the question
• May not **c**ite from the passage or uses incorrect examples/general references	• Limited examples cited from the passage/general references from the text	• **C**ites from the passage, but examples may not be as many or as strong as a shark	• **C**ites from the passage—uses strong examples as support
• Lacks elaboration	• **E**laborates somewhat	• Uses effective elaboration	• Uses strong **E**laboration
• Lacks something extra	• **S**omething extra—May attempt connection	• **S**omething extra—Has a connection	• **S**omething extra—meaningful connection

Figure 2.1

importantly, promote thinking that uses assessments for learning and assessment of learning.

Teacher's Name: <u>Chris Barbiere</u>   *Lesson:* <u> Cardiovascular Disease </u>
Unit Topic: <u> Circulatory System </u>   *Grade level:* <u> 8 </u>
BACKGROUND: CROSS-CURRICULAR Lesson with Health Unit on Fitness Training and a Healthy Heart.

Overview

Let's look at a sample lesson plan to see what a teacher planned for his or her students and then determine how assessments can be used to promote self-regulation. This unit deals with the three forms of exercise—aerobic, anaerobic, and flexibility—and how each helps maintain a healthy heart.

The students will perform each type of exercise to develop "sense" and "meaning" to the lesson while taking heart rate readings, creating statistical representations of the data, and comparing each type of exercise. The students then analyze their diet to expose the components of their diet that may lead to high cholesterol levels, obesity, and a reduction in heart health.

Essential Questions

What is healthful living?
What role does exercise play in healthful living?

Objectives

I will be able to explain and justify five of the major factors associated with cardiovascular disease.

I will be able to explain, justify, and provide solutions to reduce cardiovascular disease and create a plan to prevent the consequences of cardiovascular disease.

Demonstration of Student Learning

I will be able to compare and contrast the concept of "vascular age" between a teenager and adult and explain my rationale. I will provide suggestions for both groups to create a health plan.

Standards to Be Addressed: CCSS

HEALTH

Indicator 2.1–11: Analyze a health profile to determine strengths and potential health risks resulting from risk factors and health-enhancing behaviors.

Standard 2.1 seeks to address these concerns by supporting the concept of health promotion and disease prevention. The underlying principle of this standard is that all students need to learn to take enhancing behaviors that support lifelong wellness.

CONTENT AREA: Health
GRADE: 8

UNIT #: 1
UNIT NAME: Wellness

Table 2.1. Wellness

	Rubric for assessing student work		
Basic: needs improvement progressing	Progressing	On target	Exceeds target
No evidence to support an effective plan that will increase healthy lifestyle choices and wellness throughout a person's lifetime.	Little evidence to support an effective plan that will increase healthy lifestyle choices and wellness throughout a person's lifetime. More evidence needed to make a stronger case.	Provides some evidence to support an effective plan that will increase healthy lifestyle choices and wellness throughout a person's lifetime.	Consistently provides evidence to support an effective plan that will increase healthy lifestyle choices and wellness throughout a person's lifetime.

Readiness Set: Eight to Ten Minutes

Teacher will pose several questions to the students to promote stimulation of prior knowledge. The teacher will be mindful of the student responses when a student answers the three questions so as to determine which students will need additional help during independent practice time.

Students note their answers to questions:

1. *What do you know about heart attacks? (A question to develop meaning and to make sense of the assignments by tying in the student frame of reference)*
2. *Do you know anyone who had a heart attack or have you ever seen someone have a heart attack on a television show? If you did, what happened? (Question to determine baseline information from the student to provide data to the teacher to be able to tier the lesson)*
3. *Tell your neighbor why exercise is good for a health heart. Please share what exercise you do to stay healthy.* (Cross-Curricular of Science and Health) *(This activity will help promote student discussion and also help the students see a relationship between heart attack and the exercise and ties in Science and Health.)*

Students will pair–share their information to discuss the three questions that were posed. The discussion may evolve into students reporting that they know folks who exercise and still have heart attacks.

The teacher will expand the lesson by providing information that identifies other benefits as a result of participating in regular physical activity.

- *Did you know that physical activity boosts mental wellness?* Participating in regular physical activity can relieve tension, anxiety, depression, and anger. You may not only notice a "feel good sensation" immediately following your physical activity, but most people also note an improvement in general well-being over time during the weeks and months as physical activity becomes a part of your daily routine. The teacher will talk about the reason why one feels good after exercising.
- *Did you know you can learn better in school if you participate in physical activity?* Exercise increases the flow of oxygen which directly affects the brain. Your mental acuity and memory can be improved with physical activity.
- *Did you know that physical activity can make you healthier?* Physical activity improves your physical wellness. It strengthens your immune system and decreases the risk of developing heart diseases and cancer.
- *Did you know physical activity can prolong your optimal health?* Without regular physical activity, the body slowly loses its strength, stamina, and ability to function well. For each hour you participate in physical activity, you'll gain about two hours of additional life expectancy.

For students who have actually seen someone have a heart attack, they will have a vivid memory of the experience and they may be emotionally charged compare to students who have only seen a heart attack by an actor on television. The students who have actually seen a heart attack will be able to describe in detail what they experienced.

Cross-curricular questions are tied to the realization of heart attacks and exercise with the belief the exercise helps to prevent heart attacks. Hopefully, the discussion will also include healthy living and eating in conjunction with exercise.

The following is a list of suggested websites:

- The American Heart Association

  http://www.heart.org/kids

- Physical Activity and the Health of Young People

  (Centers for Disease Control and Prevention)
  http://www.cdc.gov/healthyyouth/physicalactivity/facts.htm

- Nutrition and Health of Young People

  http://www.cdc.gov/healthyyouth/nutrition/facts.htm

- How Much Sleep Do I Need?

  http://www.cdc.gov/sleep/about_sleep/how_much_sleep.htm about two hours of additional life expectancy

READINESS SET

The teacher will ask the students to place their hand over their heart to feel it beating. After they feel it beating, the teacher will have them work in pairs to listen to their heart. They will use two different instruments to measure their heart beat. One instrument will be the Adult Kit with Stethoscope, and the other instrument will be a monitor with Auto Inflating to allow each child to hear his or her own heartbeat and that of another classmate.

Making Sense and Meaning Activity

Explain that the sound they hear means that the heart (a pump) is pumping blood throughout the body. Explain that blood carries oxygen to all parts of the body. (Incorporate the respiratory system into the discussion for an interdisciplinary approach to the topic.) Once the class has established that the heart is a pump, the next step is to understand that the heart is also a muscle.

Ask the class, "how do you keep your muscles in shape and strong"? The class will determine that exercise keeps the heart strong and that realization will enable students to conclude that the heart, like other muscles, needs exercise. Ask the students what they do to keep their muscles in shape.

Ask the class what happens when they exercise Someone will say that their heartbeat accelerates. Some students may even have a smartwatch or fitbit which can monitor blood pressure so they are aware of their blood pressure all the time. Ask the class if they would conclude that exercise for the body is also exercise for the heart. The goals is to make the connection that exercise for the body is exercise for the heart and explain how exercise helps the heart to pump more effectively.

Brainstorm other ways to keep the heart healthy and list them on the board. At some point in the discussion, students will mention nutrition, healthy eating, healthy life style, as well as exercise. During this exercise, the teacher will list keywords on the board so they can be used for a homework assignment.

The consolidation for closure activity will be to ask the students to use the information from the class and their research to determine how they keep healthy. They will complete the sentence, "I keep my heart healthy by . . . " and write their answers on a 3 × 5 index card and submit it to the teacher at the end of the period. This activity will be the consolidation for closure activity. It will also be used for an entrance ticket into the classroom. Students can get into groups based on what they do to keep their heart healthy. For example, those students who run to for a health heart will be one group; students who do yoga will be a second group; students who eat health will be a third group.

Addressing Learning Styles

The tactile learners can create a puzzle that includes the bodyparts being discussed or can use heart models.

The auditory learners can listen to teacher-selected podcasts.

After the Readiness Set is introduced, the Demonstration of Student Learning (DSL) is explained to the class. The teacher can tell the class, "To ensure that I know you have learned the concepts being taught, you will be asked to compare and contrast two people's age and exercise level and asked to create a health plan for each group."

Demonstration of Student Learning

"I will be able to compare and contrast the 'vascular age' between a teenager and an adult and justify how exercise can help prevent cardiovascular disease in any person."

To help the students self-regulate, the teacher will share with the class a sample action plan that is an example of an exemplar and the rubric which they used to assess the assignment so students can self-regulate their own learning. Students will be encouraged to promote an action plan that is research-based.

Instructional Input Stage

Modeling (five minutes): Students will create an action plan to help prevent cardiovascular disease from becoming a serious health problem. The purpose of the action plan is having the students demonstrate their knowledge of the concept. They will be encouraged to self-regulate their learning by setting benchmarks which they can use for short- and long-term goals.

The students are told to use the rubrics to self-monitor. Students will also be asked to show evidence of how they used the rubric. Students may present their action plan in any appropriate format: written account, song, poem/short story, blog, wikispace, play, SMART board file, PowerPoint, video, radio interview, and the like. The critical factor is that the students will be taught to use self-regulation learning strategies throughout the lesson.

Large-Group Activity

The teacher will provide information to the students about heart disease and the value of exercise. After the large-group instruction activity, small groups of three to four students will be selected and the groups will be predetermined. They will include students who have varied multiple intelligences so they can use the strength of each "intelligence."

Small-Group Activity

Students will work in small groups for approximately twenty minutes to read and discuss three articles. While they are in the small groups, the teacher will ask students questions to determine if they are on track or off track in their thinking and if everyone is participating in the small group.

The students will use a jigsaw approach in that each student will have one article to read after which they will share information from the article with the remaining students in their group. There will be a list of clarifying questions students can use during this activity.

Activities (twenty minutes): Students will work in groups to discuss different resources.

1. Articles

    Exercise and Cardiovascular Health | *Circulation*
    circ.ahajournals.org/content/107/1/e2

2. Internet

    The American Heart Association
    http://www.heart.org/kids
    Physical Activity and the Health of Young People
    (Centers for Disease Control and Prevention)
    http://www.cdc.gov/healthyyouth/physicalactivity/facts.htm
    Nutrition and Health of Young People
    http://www.cdc.gov/healthyyouth/nutrition/facts.htm
    How Much Sleep Do I Need?
    http://www.cdc.gov/sleep/about_sleep/how_much_sleep.htm about two hours of additional life expectancy.

3. Research Journals
    http://scholar.google.com/scholar?q=cardiovascular+health+journals&hl=en&as_sdt=0&as_vis=1&oi=scholart&sa=X&ved=0ahUKEwir2onm8bjTAhVE6iYKHX_PDckQgQMILDAA

Activities are assigned or differentiated for individuals based on their reading level. To help differentiate the lesson, there are various programs that can provide leveled reading texts so all the students can read the same article if they choose. Students keep in mind the Essential Question while reading. Early finishers will have anchor activities to pursue.

During the small-group activity, teacher will monitor the group activity. Teacher will ask probing questions as well as reflective questions to ensure that the students are staying focused on the task at hand as well as obtaining information necessary for them to do their report.

The teacher may say: "As you pair–share your ideas about heart attacks, exercise, and healthy heart, who can share with me what was discussed?" During the discussion, the teacher will refer back to the student learning target objective to keep the students focused. "Don't forget today we are learning about the heart, heart disease, and exercise."

The teacher can also remind students: "Today you are learning about heart disease and exercise and you will be held responsible for comparing and contrasting information. You will need to collect details and facts to be able to justify your answers." During the small-group activity, students will be encouraged to self-regulate their learning.

Check for Understanding

Teacher circulates throughout class and uses targeted questioning and graphic organizer checklist to check for individual understanding. As students are reading the articles, the teacher will ask: "what is the most important concept in the article and why?" Or, the teacher can do a "quick write" and ask the students to summarize what they read in one minute. The teacher will review what they have written in order to determine if the students are extracting the critical elements of the paper.

Assessments

Formative assessment: Completion of closure activity and exit cards on the major theme of the day. Formative assessment will involve the muddiest point, quick write, "I would like to know more about . . . ," or "Cloudy Points," "Tell Me More," or "Blog."

Guided Practice and Monitoring of Small Groups (Fifteen)

Students read the article and use the graphic organizer provided to summarize the important points. Anchor charts, rubrics, exemplars, informational charts, and reference charts will be available for self-regulation.

To further self-regulation, the learning environment will have heart models for students to examine. Those students who are tactile and visual learners will have models available for their examination.

Students will meet in groups to discuss their articles and complete a chart listing the similar information contained in all of the articles. The students will determine three most important points from their research which may be used to answer the Essential Questions posed.

Students will be asked to discuss the following in their groups:

1. How did the research help with your understanding of the Health Unit on Exercise? Why? What do you not agree with from your evidence and why? Please cite evidence to justify your response.
2. What evidence will you cite to describe "vascular age" as it refers to cardiovascular health?
3. What self-regulation strategies did you use during this activity?

Teacher circulates around the room to question the students to promote their metacognition and guides the discussion with higher-level questions involving analysis, synthesis, and evaluation. The teacher will also use checks for understanding techniques of singling, sampling, or choral responses.

There will be a class discussion on the major points the students found in the research and how this information may help students create their action plan. Signaling and sampling to check for understanding will enable the teacher to determine if the students have the main concepts or if instruction is needed.

Other examples of checks of understanding can include strategies listed in Table 2.2.

Table 2.2. Other examples of checks of understanding

Strategy	Example
1. Hand Signals: Thumbs Up/Down;	The teacher asks students to display a hand signal to indicate their understanding.
2. Three, Two, One Finger	• I understand and can explain it (e.g., *thumbs up or three fingers*).
	• I do not yet understand (e.g., *thumbs down or one finger*).
	• I'm not completely sure (e.g., *thumb sideways or two fingers*).
3. Whiteboard	The teacher asks the students a question during the lesson
	• Students have time to process the question and write responses on the whiteboard.
	• Students hold up the whiteboards and display their answers.
	• The teacher checks the whiteboards for student answers. If many students have the correct answer, the teacher can have students with the correct answer talk to students who have the incorrect answers. If everyone has a correct answer, the teacher can read the answer and ask everyone if they agree. Since students may not be able to see all the whiteboards, they will hear the choral response and determine that their answer is the correct answer.
	• The teacher restates the correct answer with the whole class.
	• Since not everyone can see all the whiteboards, the teacher must be mindful of sharing information with the whole class so they hear the correct answers and so they know that they are "on track."

(Continued)

46   Chapter 2

Table 2.2   (Continued)

Strategy	Example
4. Tell Me What You Know	Students summarize in one minute the main ideas they got from the class during the small-group discussion or after the teachers review the choral responses.
	The students can review their one-minute summary with their classmates as it would be an effective strategy for students to engage in dialogue and metacognition.
5. Cloudy Point	Students write about the point they had the most difficulty understanding during the lesson. Or, students can tell their partner what they had difficulty with during the lesson.
	Bright Point: Student can write or say what they enjoyed most about the information they gathered during the small-group activity or from the large-group lesson. This information can lead to discussions, justifications of responses, debates, pros/cons, or other kinds of activities.
6. I Have a Question; Who Has the Answer?	Students who have a muddy point can raise a question for a classmate to answer.

The whole purpose of the checking for understanding is to monitor the student learning to adjust the instruction based on the information received from the monitoring.

Activities to Promote Checks for Understanding

The natural flow of feedback from the checks for understanding would promote student engagement activities and differentiation of the lessons. For example, one activity a teacher can do to collect information and engage students is *agree/disagree*. Teachers can have students who agree find a classmate who disagrees to have a discussion. The activity can also involve physical activity as all the students who agree stand in a straight line. Students who disagree will form a line facing the students in the agree line. The task is to have each line try to recruit members form the other team. The team with the greatest gains, i.e. the agree line had 7 students at the start of the activity and wound up with 10 students had a gain of 3. If disagree had 7 students to start and wound up with 4, they lost.

The teacher can also engage the students by having them develop pros and cons to the comments made. From the pros and cons, debate teams can be formed.

As the lesson reaches its conclusion, the teacher asks students to develop student-generated test questions which will be used as a test or quiz. Students will submit their questions to the teachers. The teacher will review all the submissions to determine what the students feel is important enough to be on a test.

The teacher can also use the review questions to develop a four-corners activity. Students can strongly agree, agree, disagree, or strongly disagree and can go to one of the four corners to vote on how they feel. They can have a discussion with their colleagues while at the corner to determine if their opinion still remains the same. While they are in their four corners, students can list of all the reasons for their voting.

The next step would be to have the strongly agree and agree confirm and come up with a list of phrases to capture their major points. The strongly agree/agree team can meet with the strongly disagree/disagree team to share their findings. Each team can make a list of questions to be used for a homework assignment. Students will be required to develop a definition and justification for the focus work. Students will bring in their list of questions the next day as an entrance "ticket" to class. The teacher will select the best questions to use for the quiz.

Closing the Lesson

After the instructional delivery stage, teacher will do a consolidation for closing activity. Many closing activities that can be used include the following:

1. *"Hot listing."* Students give the teacher a list of keywords and concepts from the lesson.
2. *Tell Me What You Know; Summary.* Students write a short summary of what they learned and give it to the teacher on their way out of the class which then becomes their "exit ticket."
3. *"Twitter summary."* Students capture the essence of the lesson by writing what they learned in one sentence.
4. *Big-concept map.* Based on the lesson, students diagram the relationships of the concepts that were taught. In the center of the map is the essential concept with supporting ideas surrounding the big concept.
5. *Pro and con grid.* Students make a "T"-chart and write down the pros and cons of the concepts taught.
6. *Three-column chart*: "What I know, what I want to know, what I learn" could be one heading. Another version would be "What, so what, now what" or "What I knew, what I know now, what I still don't know."
7. *Exit ticket or "ticket to leave."* Students summarize what they learned on a 3 × 5 index card.
8. Finally, students can show what they know by developing a product using multiple intelligences.

USING MULTIPLE INTELLIGENCES AS A DOL

Students can select an appropriate intelligence to use as a DOL:

Linguistic:

Develop an inventive dialogue between a teenager and a senior citizen about healthy habits.
Have students lead a class discussion.
Students will use research to create a point of view for a ten-minute class presentation. They will also have handouts for classmates to use based on their research.
Students will write in their journal an essay on health that will be reviewed by the teacher the next day.

Logical–Mathematical:

Students will research articles about cardiovascular disease statistics and graph or plot the information.
Students will develop a graph and explain the graph to the class.
Students will create word or math puzzles related to cardiovascular disease.

Musical:

Students will create a rap song about "The Healthy Heart" or about developing a healthy heart plan.
Students will choose their action plan and create a song or video about good health, exercise, or healthy heart practices.
Students will use GarageBand to create a song about exercise and nutrition.
Students will create a podcast based on the information they researched. They will write a short description about the podcast to "advertise" it.

Bodily Kinesthetic:

Students will create an interpretive dance whose story line is about a healthy heart.
Students will create an activity about the heart or a play about the heart that they act out.

Spatial–Visual:

Students will create a graphic organizer about exercise and nutrition for a healthy heart.

Students will construct a graphic model about a healthy heart or exercise.
Students will develop a mind map for a healthy heart.

Interpersonal:

Students will create a script for an interview between a reporter and heart expert.
Students will create a FAQ list about nutrition based on information from interviewing fellow students.
Students will work in pairs on a "newspaper" article on what they learned that day.
Students will develop a board game for the class.

Intrapersonal:

Students will write a paragraph on what the lesson meant to them and provide advice to a friend based on their research.
Student will make entries into their daily journal and what they will do to promote a healthy heart.

Naturalist:

Students will create their own case study based on the lesson tied to exercise and the value of organic food for a healthy heart.
Students will compare and contrast two articles related to the environment.
Students will write about the value of organic foods on health.

Accommodations

- Teacher will provide differentiated reading assignments and provide articles based on the student's reading level.
- Teacher will make recorded passages for students who are auditory learners.
- Teacher will provide different levels of graphic organizers for students with IEPs.
- Small-group instruction or one-to-one time will be utilized for individualized attention.

Assessments

Formative assessment. Formative assessments will be done during the lesson via checks for understandings and at the end of the lesson via a completion of closure activity using exit cards.

Consolidation for Closure: (10 minutes)

Students reflect on the following questions:

1. How did today's lesson help me in the construction of my action plan?
2. What did I learn and how will it apply in tomorrow's lesson?
3. How will I answer the Essential Question based on what I learned today?
4. How will I describe what I learned today using the assignment rubric to assess my lesson?

Teacher will ask students to use an exit ticket to answer one of the aforementioned four questions (overt closure). After the students answer the questions, they will discuss their answers with their partner/group (covert closure).

Independent Practice

Students continue with the formulation of their action plan at home and must have one component of the plan completed by the next day. Students will come to class the next day with an "Admit Ticket" in which they will list any questions, concerns, barriers they had while doing their homework. The admit slip will be collected by the teachers as students enter class. The teacher will read the slips aloud. The teacher will then begin the lesson based on what was read to the class.

Once the lesson plan is developed, there are two distinct approaches to using assessments. One approach is to use assessments for learning at the end (summative), and the other way is to use assessments for learning during the class (formative).

ASSESSMENTS FOR LEARNING

The teacher must be aware of the student's progress during the lesson and adjust accordingly. Using formative assessments should help determine what the students have mastered, what they still need, and what needs to happen next.

Strategies for assessing student progress can be done overtly or covertly, individually or collectively. For assessments to be overt, the teacher will employ several different modalities as students may be visual, auditory, or tactile learners.

For the visual learners, the students may draw something to show what they know, use a concept map, complete a Venn diagram, or use portable whiteboards. Students will synthesize information that they are learning and then graphically represent what you have learned to teach.

For the tactile learners, students will share notes during the instruction. Students can highlight specific passages or make a list of keywords from their notes to use as a study guide.

For the auditory learners, students can turn it and talk, pair–share, or work in a small group to discuss their findings. They will share information with the rest of the class.

Once a student's progress via various learning styles is assessed, the next consideration is: will the assessments be done via a spaced or distributed approach?

ASSESSMENTS: SPACED OR DISTRIBUTED?

The important fact to remember is that an effective teacher enhances a student's learning. Researcher S. Paul Wright, Sandra Horn, and William Sanders (1997) made the following observation from a study they conducted involving 60,000 students in grades three through five:

> The results of the study will document that the most important factor affecting student learning is the teacher. In addition, the results show wide variation in effectiveness among teachers. The immediate and clear implication is that work can be done to prove education by improving the effectiveness among teachers than any other single factor. Effective teachers appeared to be effective with students of all achievement levels, regardless of the level of heterogeneity in the classroom. If the teacher is ineffective, students on the teacher's tutelage will show inadequate progress academically regardless of how similar or different they are regarding their academic achievement. (63)

The logical question is, what do effective teachers do for students with varied abilities? The answer provided by research is that they have well-planned lessons, starting with objectives, Essential Questions, effective classroom management, communicate learning goals, plan cooperative activities, practice activities, use of quiz and prompts, and student involvement (Hattie 1992; Marzano, Marzano, and Pickering 2003; Marzano, Pickering, and Pollock 2001). All this data helps to differentiate the lesson to meet student's individual needs. Inherent in the process is the use of formative assessments because formative assessments provide important data to teachers to use for differentiation of instruction. Specifically, the research on formative assessments was:

Paul Black and Dylan Uilian (1998) describe how effective assessments can be:

> The research reported here shows conclusively that formative assessments improves learning. The gains in achievements appear to be considerable, and as noted earlier amongst the largest ever reported for educational interventions. . . . If scores could be achieved on a nationwide scale, it would be

equivalent to raising the mathematics attainment score of an average country like England, New Zealand, or the United States into the top five after the Pacific rim countries Singapore, Korea, Japan and Hong Kong. (61)

The assessment process begins with the student learning target (objective) to identify what the student must know and the assessment will cause a student to show the teacher or demonstrate to the teacher what they know by providing evidence, that is, a DSL.

From School-Dependent or Teacher Dependent to Self-Dependent

In all cases, the student will be demonstrating to the teacher that he or she can apply what was taught. The focus of learning shifts from the student being a consumer (what he or she is expected to learn today) to a producer (apply what he or she learned). The mental shift is from what I am doing during a lesson to what I will be doing after lesson. The shift is from learning a skill (a learning activity) to developing mastery of a skill or moving from passive learning to active learning (a learning outcome).

The shift in thinking is a mind-set shift regarding the role of assessment. The shift is releasing the student from one who is a "school-dependent learner" to become a self-regulating learner or a self-dependent learner. This type of learning is a shift from students relying on the teacher (school-dependent learner) to student learning (empowerment) to the student relying on himself or herself to seek knowledge (self-dependent). The process for self-dependent requires student self-regulation.

In the school-dependent process, the instructional focus is what must be taught. In the school-dependent model, knowledge is provided to the learner so the learner is dependent on the teacher for acquisition of facts. In the self-dependent model, the learner is provided information (empowered) and expected to gather information that is needed so he or she can apply what is taught for the maximization of learning. The effort is to connect the student's culture, language, and cognition into a schema whereby the student is not school-dependent or waiting for the teacher to tell him or her what to do or how to think.

Shifting the Mind-Set to Becoming Self-Dependent

The shift toward self-regulation for self-dependency begins with the tailoring of the students' lesson in addition to teaching students the self-regulation strategies. It is the use of formative assessments to collect data to use for differentiating the student learning.

There are two important considerations for the teacher to be mindful throughout the lesson: one, to use frequent checks of understanding and, two, provide timely and constructive feedback to students while encouraging them to succeed.

The failure to provide feedback or having limited feedback along the way will not provide the guidance that students need; otherwise, the students may presume that they are doing well. Additionally, feedback is needed so students continue to try. Students who do not receive any feedback during a lesson or after doing a task tend to rate themselves higher on their achievement. It is the feedback that enables the students to assess how well they are doing on a test.

Attribution Theory

Encouraging students to do well is one aspect of the attribution theory. Attribution theory postulates that the manner in which students explain or attribute failure and/or success will encourage or discourage them. The other attributes include the ability, will, and task difficulty.

Of all the attributes, effort is the most encouraging because:

- Students who are told they made good effort are inclined to work harder for future exams. More importantly, the teacher can share with the student strategies to use for improvement and that it requires more effort, so the student will be inclined to try the strategies.
- The downside to praising only effort is that the students will become discouraged if they worked hard and did not get the desired results.
- Encouraging students who did well and worked hard will promote their self-esteem.
- Every coach knows that success gets success. Once the students experience success, they will be eager for more success so encouraging students to try hard is the preferred strategy. If they tried hard and were not successful, the feeling of pride in knowing that they tried their best will offset the guilt they may feel if they fail.
- Stressing effort implies that the student worked to achieve a desired result as opposed to being "lucky" and getting the desired result. Productive struggle is in line with the new mathematical practices of persevering in problem-solving. Teachers can help to modulate a student's effort as opposed to luck.

It's not unusual to see elementary teachers give stickers or prizes to students who try hard for an activity. Additionally, teachers will give students words of encouragement to help them to try harder on the next assignment. Intuitively, teachers are encouraging students to continue to try hard so they will become successful and feel good about what they have accomplished as a result of their effort. What are some other ways for assessments to help students?

COGNITIVE STRATEGIES IN ENHANCING LEARNING

Roediger and Pye identify three general principles that are very inexpensive to employ and enhance cognitive strategies to improve student learning. The research, examined by Dunlosky, Rawson, Marsh, Nathan, and Willingham, examined ten promising strategies to improve learning. Dunlosky et al. concluded that five strategies were useful.

The Magic Three Strategies for Cognition

From those five strategies, there are three general principles:

1. Massed practice is different than distribution (spacing and interleaving) and has an advantage. Use massed practice for short-term learning and distributed practice for long-term learning.
2. Use frequent assessment of learning (direct and indirect positive effects of quizzing and testing) and checks for understanding to assess student comprehension of learning.
3. Have students seek meaning by asking why questions, explanatory questioning (elaborate interrogation and self-explanation) as it helps to promote their metacognition.

Let's see how the three principles can be applied to assessment beginning with distribution.

Use massed practice the day before a test as the learning will be short term. Distribution addresses the concept of spacing and interleaving material as well as a strategy to use for long-term learning. Distribution can also be practiced as a learning strategy for the student to use while doing homework.

The general notion is that practice makes permanent, so practice for perfection. The practice of repeating a task over and over again is one way to learn and is referred to as mass or blocked practice.

Interleaving

The other way to learn information would be to space the practice or to "interleave" the material. Using the process of interleaving, the information is spaced over time and done in smaller chunks. Over a period of time, the learning and the material is intermixed.

Another example of interleaving would be to have problems for the students to do, followed by problems that are already completed, so students can see the correct answers to the problems. The effects of spacing material are effective over a period of time as opposed to studying the day or night before a test, which is known as cramming.

Cramming

Cramming before a test can result in short-term success; however, it still not be effective strategy for long term learning. Cramming and rushing through readings are not ideal ways to feel ready for any academic challenge. Teachers often tell students that all the caffeine and energy drink in the world to stay up the night before a test is not the best way to study as it does not make effective use of time or develop effective study habits for self-regulation.

In fact, after going through the experience of cramming and skimming texts, one may find the anxiety experienced while trying to catch up on a semester, or entire school year is just too stressful and not worth it. Having students remember how it feels the next time testing rolls around will help the student see the value of being better prepared.

Sometimes teachers would hear a student who studied the night before a test say, "Don't bump into me as all the information may fall out." Who among us has not studied the night before a test and actually did well on the test? And if you did do well, how did you feel after the test?

Spacing versus Cramming

A more effective way to study would be to space the learning over time. The student can begin studying months before exam. After the initial study session, the student can take a break for a week and then come back and study.

Spacing concept can also be applied by the teacher during the period of instructional delivery. It is the concept of "prime time/downtime and primary/recent." Prime time/downtime and primacy/recency was written about by Sousa (2000, 2001). He based his work on the research done by Ebbinghaus (1885). The basic premise is that students will remember information that is done at the beginning of a class period, which is referred to as prime time.

Students will also remember information that is presented at the end of a period, which is referred to as recency. Therefore the approach is to introduce information at the beginning of a class period (prime time 1), then students can work on the information for a period of time (downtime), with the last part of the class period, teachers can use for prime time again (prime time 2). During the "downtime" activity, teachers can assess the student progress.

As the assessments are done, the teacher can establish skill groups based on the targeted instruction during the independent learning time or during guided practice. It is during the guided practice that the teacher questions the students to determine the depth of their knowledge regarding their understanding what must be done. Teacher can also encourage the students self-monitor or self-regulate their learning.

Strategies for Massed or Distributed Learning

In summary, there are strategies to employ for massed or distributed learning:

- Use massed learning strategies for short-term test-taking (the next day, as in cramming the day before a test). Use distributed learning for long-term learning. If the test is a week away, space the learning a few days apart. If the learning is a month away, space the learning a week after the initial trial.
- Both massed or distributed learning can use interleaving. The process of interleaving involves having problems for student to solve and interleaving the problems with problems that are already solved. So one process involves the student solving problems while the other process involves the student explaining the process.
- Use various modalities of visual with auditory or tactile with auditory. If possible have students incorporate graphics, visuals, or multiple representations in their problem-solving.
- Connect and integrate abstract and concrete representations of concepts; multiple representations of concrete representations help make the abstract concepts easy to understand.
- Use assessments to promote learning; make assessments to your friends and not your foe. Formative assessment and quizzes promote learning.

Strategies to Use for Interleaving Include

Ways to implement interleaving:

- Have the students do a few examples, then have one example worked out for the students so they can refer back to it.
- Have examples completed for students so they could see exactly what must be done. In this manner, the students can start to self-regulate what they are doing.
- Use interleaving in the classroom during student-independent work time. One way for this to occur would be for students to present the answers to their tablemate.
- After the students spend X amount of time working on their project, they can turn to their neighbor in explaining what they have done.

- Give a tablemate the answers to a problem which they can check to see if the students did the work correctly.
- Call upon students to explain their process; any person at the table can assess their work, with the student explaining the process. This format would be a viable alternative as only one student is doing the work while the remaining students are checking that work.
- Have students work in pairs so that they are doing more of the discussion.

Strategies for Formative Assessments

- Use student self-explanation and elaborative interrogation. The purpose of this activity is to ensure that the student begins to develop a deeper understanding why something is occurring and can articulate the reasons for his or her answer.
- Have students self-explain when they are doing an assignment and justify why they use the various methods during the course of the assignment.
- Use questions to determine how well they can explain what they are doing. The driving concept for student talk is that students are beginning to develop metacognition as well as self-regulation.
- Use student conferences.
- Have students keep a journal of what they learn during the class period which the teacher can then review at a later date.
- Uses quizzes. A quick quiz given during a lesson will provide feedback to the teacher on what the students retained and what needs to be re-taught.

Hopefully, the use of test and quizzes will prompt the students to engage in more self-testing if they see the advantage of this methodology of using tests for learning. Students will quickly realize that self-testing will enable them to see what they need to study, what they understand, what the next steps are for more effective comprehension.

In the next chapter, we will discuss closing a lesson.

BIBLIOGRAPHY

Caine, R. N., and G. Caine. 1990. "Understanding a Brain Based Approach to Learning and Teaching." *Educational Leadership* 48 (2): 66–70.
———. 1991. *Making Connections: Teaching and the Human Brain*. Alexandria, VA: Association for Supervision and Curriculum Development.
Caine, R. N., G. Caine, C. McClintic, and K. Klimek. 2004. *12 Brain/Mind Learning Principles in Action: The Fieldbook for Making Connections, Teaching, and the Human Brain*. Thousand Oaks, CA: Corwin Press.

Carpenter, S. K., and E. L. Delosh. 2005. "Application of the Testing and Spacing Effects to Name Learning." *Applied Cognitive Psychology* 19 (5): 619–36.

———. 2006. "Impoverished Cue Support Enhances Subsequent Retention: Support for the Elaborative Retrieval Explanation of the Testing Effect." *Memory & Cognition* 34: 268–76.

Carpenter, Shana K., and Harold Pashler. 2007. "Testing beyond Words: Using Tests to Enhance Visuospatial Map Learning." *Psychonomic Bulletin & Review* 14: 215–35.

Carpenter, Shana K., H. Pashler, and E. Vul. 2006. "What Types of Learning Are Enhanced by a Cued Recall Test?" *Psychonomic Bulletin & Review* 13: 826–30.

Carpenter, Shana K., Harold Pashler, John T. Wixted, and Edward Vul. 2008. "The Effects on Learning and Forgetting." *Memory & Cognition* 36 (2): 438.

DuFour, Richard, DuFour, Rebecca, Eaker, Robert, Karhanek, Gayle. 2004. *Whatever It Takes: How Professional Learning Communities Respond When Kids Don't Learn*. Bloomington, IN: National Educational Service.

Ebbinghaus, H. 1885. Memory: A contribution to Experimental Psychology, translated by Henry A Ruger and Clare E. Bussenius (1913) originally published in New York by Teachers College in the History of Psychology, as internet resource developed by Christopher D. Green, New Your University, Toronto, Ontario.

Fisher, D., and N. Frey. 2007. *Checking for Understanding: Formative Assessment Techniques for Your Classroom*. Alexandria, VA: Association for Supervision and Curriculum Development.

Guttentag, R. H. 1984. "The Mental Effort Requirement of Cumulative Rehearsal: A Developmental Study." *Journal of Experimental Child Psychology* 37: 92–106.

Hattie, J. Measuring the Effects of Schooling (1992). *Australian Journal of Education*, Volume: 36 issue: 1, page(s): 5–13 Issue published: April 1, 1992 https://doi.org/10.1177/000494419203600102.

Higbee, Kenneth. 2001. *Your Memory How It Works and How to Improve It*. Englewood Cliffs, NJ: Prentice Hall.

Marzano, R. J., Pickering, D. J., and Pollock, J. E. 2001. *Classroom instruction that works Research-based strategies for increasing student achievement*. Alexandria, VA ASCD.

Marzano, R. J., Marzano, J.S. and Pickering, D. J. 2003. Association for Supervision and Curriculum Development 1703 N. Beauregard St. Alexandria, VA 22311-1714 USA.

Marzano, Robert. 2006. *Classroom Assessment and Grading That Work*. Alexandria, VA: Association for Supervision and Curriculum Development.

Pashler, H., P. Bain, B. Bottge, A. Graesser, K. Koedinger, M. McDaniel, and J. Metcalfe. 2007. *Organizing Instruction and Study to Improve Student Learning* (NCER 2007–2004). Washington, DC: National Center for Education Research, Institute of Education Sciences, US Department of Education. http://ncer.ed.gov.

Pressley, M., and P. Beardel-Dinary. 1992. "Memory Strategy Instruction That Promotes Good Instruction Process." In *Memory Improvement: Implications for Memory Theory*, ed. D. Hermann, H. Meingartner, and A. Searleman, 79–100. New York: Springer-Verlag.

Roediger, H. L., and J. D. Karpicke. 2006a. "The Power of Testing Memory: Basic Research and Implications for Educational Practice." *Perspectives on Psychological Science* 1 (3): 181–210.

———. 2006b. "Test-Enhanced Learning: Taking Memory Tests Improves Long-Term Retention." *Psychological Science* 17 (3): 249–255.

Roediger, H. L., and M. A. Pyc. 2012a. "Applying Cognitive Psychology to Education: Complexities and Prospects." *Journal of Applied Research in Memory and Cognition* 1 (4): 263–65.

———. 2012b. "Inexpensive Techniques to Improve Education: Applying Cognitive Psychology to Enhance Educational Practice." *Journal of Applied Research in Memory and Cognition* 1 (4): 242–48.

Slamecka, N. J., and P. Graf. 1978. "The Generation Effect: Delineation of a Phenomenon." *Journal of Experimental Psychology: Human Learning and Memory* 4 (6): 592–604.

Sousa, David. 2000. *How the Brain Learns*. Thousand Oaks, CA: Corwin Press.

Sousa, David. 2001. *How the Brain Learns*. Second Edition. Thousand Oaks, CA: Corwin Press.

Sousa, David. 2001. *How the Special Needs Brain Learns*. Thousand Oaks, CA: Corwin Press.

Stiggins, Rick, and J. Chappuis. 2005. "Using Student-Involved Classroom Assessment to Close Achievement Gaps." *Theory into Practice* 44 (1): 11–18.

William L. Sanders, S. Paul Wright, and Sandra P. 1997. Horn Teacher and Classroom Context Effects on Student Achievement: Implications for Teacher Evaluation, Journal of Personnel Evaluation in Education, Volume 11, Number 1, Page 57.

Woloshyn, V. E., T. Willoughby, E. Wood, and M. Pressley. 1990. "Elaborative Interrogation Facilitates Adult Learning of Factual Paragraphs." *Journal of Educational Psychology* 82 (3): 513–24.

Wood, E., M. Pressley, and P. H. Winne. 1990. "Elaborative Interrogation Effects in Children's Learning of Factual Content." *Journal of Educational Psychology* 82 (4): 741–48.

Chapter 3

Consolidation for Closure

FOCUS OF THE CHAPTER

What does brain research about the learner say relative to closing a lesson will be explored. There will also be strategies a teacher can use for closure. More importantly, strategies a student can employ to regulate or modulate their learning when not in school will be provided.

INTRODUCTION

Closure is done at the end of a lesson and it involves the student summarizing what they learned. This provides valuable insights to the teacher to use for planning subsequent lessons. Closure can be done during a lesson but it is most commonly done at the end of a lesson. What research says about closure and overt or covert closure strategies for visual, auditory, tactile, or kinesthetic learners will be provided.

Probing Questions

1. Why is consolidation for closure done?
2. How will the students show the teacher what they learned?
3. How will the teacher use what the students learned to plan the next day lesson?
4. Can overt or cover consolidation for closure use visual, auditory, kinesthetic, or tactile strategies?

BACKGROUND

In the Learner's Brain Model, the final stage of the delivery is consolidation for closure. The Learner's Brain Model helps focus classroom teachers to direct students to learn by providing information to the students, facilitating practice with guidance, and subsequently offering independent practice to solidify the learning. In appendix D, there are rubrics that can be used for coaching.

Consolidation for Closure as the Final Step of the Model

The process is called Consolidation for Closure as the purpose is for students to consolidate the information they learned during the lesson and articulate to the teacher what they are consolidating, that is, "Today I learned. . . ." The information tells the teacher how the lesson was processed by the student. This is extremely important as information is consolidated by the brain when the student sleeps.

The teacher would want the correct information to be processed and saved while the student sleeps. Since consolidation is the last step in the teacher's lesson, it is important that the teacher is aware of what the student takes away from the lesson.

With overt closure, the student tells the teacher what he or she learned today. In this process, it is obvious what the student feels is important. This task is a little more difficult with covert closure as the student is writing what he or she has learned. The teacher may not see the comments until after the student leaves, that is, as exit ticket. The teacher will have to follow up with the student the next day, and the exit ticket becomes an "entrance ticket' as it begins the discussion in the beginning of the next class.

CONSOLIDATION FOR CLOSURE

This is the last step in a lesson and is a valuable tool. Unfortunately, it is an essential lesson plan element that many times is overlooked and skipped. It often receives "short shrifts" for a variety of reasons. Many teachers claim it is because there is just not enough time to cover everything they want to teach. Another reason closure is not done is that teachers think that review is a closure activity.

Review or Closure

In the teacher's mind, a review is closure. When a review is done, however, it is usually the teacher who is doing the talking. "Do you remember class we talked about x?" Or, the teacher may say, "Remember, we covered x last week." Unfortunately, the process of the teacher talking is not closure as it is the student who must do the talking in a closure activity.

When the teacher is doing the talking, it is simply a review or summary of the lesson. It allows the teacher an opportunity to bring together his or her ideas. A quick rule of thumb is if the teacher talks, it is review; if the student talks, it is closure. Remember, the goal is for the student to talk and share his or her ideas so as to consolidate the information.

What Is Closure?

Closure is a term from Gestalt psychology. It refers to an automatic process in our perception where we "close" incomplete figures, where we "connect the dots," or fill in the gaps. A classic example is a picture of three dots in a straight line. We tend to see a line, not three separate dots. If the three dots are in the shape of a triangle, we see the triangle, not the separate dots.

One applies the psychological process of closure when looking at the three dots whether they are in a straight line or in the shape of a triangle and formed a whole, or gestalt, out of the three dots.

Since the brain is a "pattern seeker," it looks for completeness. When closure is blocked, one feels anxiety and is motivated to try to reduce that anxiety. The mind like to form wholes, gestalts. We like to see a complete big picture. When this process is blocked, the brain will fill in the blanks to make it complete.

Closure is also an important process for the learner because the learner will summarize what has been learned and engage in the process of attaching sense and meaning to the learned information. The talk and summary by the student will provide information to the teacher who can ask clarifying questions to the student to help them see relationships and develop understanding.

CLOSURE RESEARCH

What Does Research Say about Closure?

Marzano's research on instructional design states that setting objectives and providing feedback specifically asking students to assess themselves at the end of a unit "will yield a 23 percent gain" (Marzano, Pinkering, and Pollock 2001, 83).

When a teacher asks clarifying questions to a student at the end of a lesson, the purpose of the questioning is to help the student reframe his or her thinking and/or look at his or her thinking with a fresh sense of eyes. What is even more interesting is the research done by Restak (2006) in which he describes the process of "backward framing."

He states that backward design alters an already-established memory. The definition that he cites is taken from Gerald Zaltman's text: "How customers think: what consumers recall about prior products or shopping experiences will differ from their actual experiences if marketers refer to those past experiences in positive way" (Restak 2006, 160).

The research claimed that consumers can be influenced to recall their prior experiences differently; in essence, their thinking can be reconstructed. Keeping this principle in mind, closure can be very important as the teacher uses the process during "overt" closure and asks students questions to help them clarify their thinking. Or, the teacher can use the information gathered from "covert closure" from the students to plan new lessons that will focus on developing accurate and deliberate information.

Backward Framing

The technique of applying "backward framing" to consolidation for closure would start by taking the information gathered by the teacher from the student and use it as a frame of reference of what needs to be addressed. The teacher can then plan the new lesson with the information gained by tying in the information that was previously discussed. The new lesson will introduce new bits of information, facts, and data that were not discussed in a previous lesson.

The introduction of the new material would begin the process of "backward framing" or having the students view the information from a different lens. After the new information is presented, the teacher can have discussions with the students about the new bits of information.

Restak wrote about an example of backward framing done by Kathryn Braun in which unsuspecting subjects were shown an advertisement for Disney. The ad suggested that children visiting Disneyland would shake hands with Bugs Bunny (people who know Disney know that Bugs Bunny is a Warner Bros creation and not a Disney creation). Interestingly enough about 16 percent of adults who read the ad recalled meeting Bugs Bunny during a childhood visit to Disneyland!

Consolidation for Closure Process

The critical attribute of consolidation for closure is that it is a process whereby the learner will summarize what has been learned. The student will have had time to practice and rehearse what was taught and attach sense and meaning to it. The talk and summary by the student will provide information to the teacher.

Although closure is usually done at the end of a lesson, there are various times it can be done. Specifically:

- It can be done at the beginning of a lesson to summarize the previous day's assignment and develop readiness for the new lesson.
- Unlike a "Readiness Set," which is also done at the beginning of a lesson to develop student readiness by activating prior knowledge, this activity is directly related to the previous day's lesson. For example: "Yesterday we talked about the Revolutionary War in class and you had an assignment to do for home learning." Be prepared to discuss two facts from the lesson or your homework assignment.

Procedural Closure

Procedural closure can occur during the lesson when the teacher moves from one sub-learning to the next. As the teacher is reviewing an activity in a lesson that involves procedural tasks, the teacher will do a procedural closure. This practice is common in math as students are doing procedural activities and the teacher is seeking feedback from the students.

The process begins with the teacher asking the class to pair–share with their tablemates the rules of operation that was discussed. After the discussion, the teacher asks the students to apply the rules of operation to the new problems. During the share-out, students should have a printout of the rules to ensure that they are stating the proper rules.

Consolidation Closure

Closure at the end of a lesson for consolidation is called consolidation closure. The purpose is to ensure that the students are leaving with the correct information and that is why it is called closure for consolidation. The process begins again with the planning stage based upon student information. The circle is complete.

Closure Benefits

Lesson closure has many benefits which is why teachers need to set time aside for a consolidation for closure activity. It is important for a teacher to set aside a short, concentrated time period of approximately six to eight minutes for closure whenever closure is done. This is a time for students to put together everything they learned and make sense out of what has just been taught. The teacher simply asking "Does anyone have any questions?" and students answering "no" is not closure. This process does not provide feedback to the teacher which is needed if closure is to be effective.

Closure provides important feedback for both the teacher and the student. During closure, the activity assigned to the student by the teacher provides the teacher feedback about the lesson taught. It will give the teacher an idea if additional practice time is needed, if the lesson needs to be retaught, or if it is OK to move onto the next concept. After closure, if the objective was mastered, the teacher can then make the decision to move on to a new objective. Consequently, if teachers are not making time for this important element in the lesson planning and lesson delivery, it is difficult to gauge if students understood the material and have mastered the concepts and skills set at the beginning of the lesson.

Some argue the fact that not all lesson plans should contain Consolidation for Closure. Closure is the exception because it is useful for the student and the teacher. Closure provides the students the opportunity to reflect. It gives them the chance to reflect and digest what was taught. It also provides the teacher with the data to determine if the desired learning outcome of the lesson was reached. The information from closure is needed to facilitate and enhance student accomplishment especially if the student did not understand what was taught. What are some examples of closure activities?

Some examples of closure activities include students writing a summary describing what was learned in the lesson, or making a timeline plotting the events that were discussed in class, or using an exit slip. Exit slip activities serve as a great closure activity because it provides an easy way for the teacher to assess understanding and can be quickly completed on scrap paper or on an index card. Some teachers use the "3–2–1 strategy." In the 3–2–1 strategy, students write down three things that interested them, two things they learned, and one question they have.

According to Dale's Cone of Experience, we learn 10 percent of what we read, 20 percent of what we hear, 30 percent of what we see, 40 percent of what we both see and hear, 70 percent of what is discussed with others, 80 percent of what we experience personally, and 95 percent of what we teach someone else (Pastore 2003). Based on this research, teachers should remember to provide students not only the opportunities to learn but also the opportunity to teach others. As a closing activity, one might have the students model how they solved a math equation or share how they decided on their opening sentence to their writing piece through a "think aloud" presentation.

Closure Activities

As a closing activity, one can consider using questioning techniques at the end of a lesson. One should incorporate higher-level questions, not rote recall of information questions. Using question cues is great to get meaningful answers from students. The teacher presents the question and the student is required to answer the question showing the teacher that they can assimilate the information. Possible question cues that allow the students to reflect are: "I learned x and I wonder if . . . ?" Teachers can ask: "How will you apply what was taught? How would you justify the following, based on what you learned? How might you apply what you learned today? How can you explain x, based on what you learned?"

A very popular closing activity is "throwing the ball." The teacher starts off by asking a question. Students raise their hand to answer the question. The teacher throws the ball to one student. That student gets a chance to answer the question. If he or she answers it correctly, they get to ask a question and throw the ball to another classmate, who in turn will answer that question. If the student does not answer the question correctly, then the child has to throw the ball to someone else who can answer the teacher's question. During this time, they are allowed to use their notes. This encourages students to take notes during the lesson and pay attention. Most students enjoy throwing and catching the ball; therefore, they will be more attentive during the lesson so that they can later participate in the closing activity.

Another favorite is "Fishbowl." For the "Fishbowl" closing activity, students write a question on a piece of paper or index card about the lesson. Then they form an inner and outer circle. Students face each other and share their question with one other and see if the other person can answer the question. If time permits, students can even rotate to a new partner.

"I have a letter" is another favorite. For the "I have a letter" closing activity, each child is given an index card and they design a postcard to their parents explaining the day's lesson. This is great for the creative students who enjoy drawing and coloring.

Another excellent example is the creation of an "Infomercial" that explains what they learned in class that day. For students who like using technology, this is a great activity as students develop an "infomercial" based on what they learned in class.

"Create a jingle" is great for the musically inclined students. In "Create a jingle," students create a jingle that explains the main idea or important facts of the lesson.

For social studies teachers, "What Am I?" is an excellent activity that has students create clues or riddles about the key terms and quiz each other. This activity can be done in partnerships or as a class. This activity is great as a review for a unit or chapter test.

An effective and meaningful lesson closure is "Movie review" where students critique the lesson as if it was a movie.

If teachers consistently use closure activities in their lessons, students will become accustomed to the process and will be better prepared to close the lesson. Due to the fact that students know that they will be expected to do a closing activity, it is more likely that students will be more actively engaged in the lesson and will take ownership of the material being taught. Below are examples of closing activities tied to learning styles.

Table 3.1 Overt/Covert Closure and Closure Based on Learning Styles

Overt	Covert
Tell Me in Your Own Words: Students are asked to paraphrase what they learned.	Tell a Friend: Students work in pairs and share what they learned.
Tweet: Students send a tweet to the teacher. They have to consolidate what they learned into three to five key words.	I Have an Answer, Who Has a Question? Students write a question in which the answer captures the critical component of what they learned.
Red Light, Green: for elementary student, each desk has a red or green cup. The teacher will ask who agrees with her statement to turn their green cup upside down.	Signals: Students work in teams of three and share what they learned. A spokesperson is selected for the group and they share what was discussed. The rest of the class give a thumbs-up or thumbs-down if they agree or disagree.
Brainstorm: Students share their one takeaway from the lesson and come to consensus as the critical elements of the lesson.	Thesis Statement: Students summarize what they learn and then consolidate the information into a thesis statement.
Whiteboards: Students use the whiteboard to write critical points of the lesson.	Exit Tickets: Students write on an index card what they learned from the lesson. The key takeaway points.
Think, Pair, Share: Students work in small groups, share their informaton then share it with the larger group.	Writing Conference: Students are given three questions to answer, then pair–share with a buddy what they learned. They summarize what they learned and share it with the class. The student selects one key point to write about at home.
Four Corners: Teacher list a key point to the lesson and post the key point at a corner of the room. Students select which of the four points they like and go to the particular corner of the room that has their point listed. They develop a summary statement from their small-group meeting.	Response Logs: Student write in their response log what they believe is the critical elements of the lesson. The teacher reviews the logs and gives the students feedback.

	Overt	Covert
	L & A Chart: Students write what they learned and how it can be applied.	Student Checklist: Teacher has several questions that he or she asks the students and their answers are noted on a checklist.
	Keywords: Students write keywords from the lesson.	Short Summary: Students summarize what they learn in three sentences.

Visual	Auditory	Kinesthetic	Tactile
Characteristics: Use visual materials, that is, maps, pictures; write, illustrate, read, use color graphs, flowcharts	**Characteristics:** Lectures, discussions, debates, create mnemonics	**Characteristics:** Attend labs, take frequent breaks, move, assemble collections	**Characteristics:** Use printed sources, take detailed notes, use manuals, handouts, or story starters
Use of *whiteboards* *Graphic organizers* *Mind maps* *Drawing Picture* The purpose is to have students express what they learned using a variety of modalities.	Inventive Dialogue: Three "Whats" Students respond to the following: What did you learn today? What does it mean? (How is this important? relevant? useful?) What can you do with the information? (What is the practical application of the information?)	Turn and Talk: Come to My Side Students are arranged in two lines facing one another. Students discuss main points of the lesson to try to convince members from the other line to come to their line. Four Corners: The teacher has a critical point noted on paper and posted in the four corners of the room. Students select a critical point and stand in the corner which has the point that they support.	Student Checklist: Quick Write Likert Scale Students respond to teacher-generated prompts (perhaps displayed on the overhead projector or on a permanent poster in the room). The prompts are from a difficult level to an application level 1. I can apply today's lesson in the real work. . . 2. Today's lesson makes sense to me because . . . 3. I understand today's lesson because. . . 4. I enjoyed today's lesson but I have some questions. . . 5. I found today's lesson difficult because. . .

(Continued)

Table 3.1 (Continued)

Visual	Auditory	Kinesthetic	Tactile
Concept Map: Students are given a concept map and they list the main point in the center circle.	Debate: Students develop debate question to use for a class debate.	Keyword List: Students share their ideas and make a list of keywords from the notes they took.	Share a Note: Students meet in small groups and share their notes with a partner. They discuss why they selected specific points.
Important to Me: Students work in a small group at a table. In the center of the table is a chart where students can enter key phrases. After each student enters a phrase, the groups has a discussion about the key phrases.	Watch, Look, Listen: Students work in small groups and share their information with the other members of the group. Only one person speaks, and the other students are not allowed to talk except to ask a clarifying question. After everyone has had a turn, students can engage in conversation with their team mates.	Stations: Students write a critical point on an index card and leave it on a desk in one corner of the room. The class is divided into four groups and each groups starts at a specific corner. After a group reads the notes at one corner of the room, they move to the next corner. Eventually they will circulate through the four corners.	My Summary: Students write a summary of what they learned and create a one-page note for the rest of the class.

The next chapter will talk about the role of reflection in the instructional process and for self-regulation.

Please use the Student Interview rubric in appendix C, to assess student learning.

BIBLIOGRAPHY

Center for Educational Research and Innovation. 1999. *Innovating Schools*. Paris: Organization for Economic Co-Operation and Development.

Duncan, C. A., and J. M. Clemons. 2012. "Closure: It's More Than Just Lining Up." *Strategies* 25 (5): 30–32. http://www.ingentaconnect.com/content/aahperd/strat/2012/00000025/00000005/art00007. Accessed June 24, 2012.

Fisher, Douglas, and Nancy Frey. 2004. *Improving Adolescent Literacy: Strategies at Work*. Upper Saddle River, NJ: Pearson Education.

Gardner, Howard. 2007. *Five Minds for the Future*. Boston, MA: Harvard Business School Press.
Gozzi, Raymond. 2003. "Seeking Closure." *ECT: A Review of General Semantics* 60 (3): 295.
Marzano, R. J. 2007. *Instructional Practices That Work*. Alexandria, VA: Association for Supervision and Curriculum Development.
Marzano, R. L., D. J. Pinkering, and J. E. Pollock. 2001. *Classroom Instruction That Works: Research-Based Strategies for Increasing Student Achievement*. Alexandria, VA: Association for Supervision and Curriculum Development.
Pastore, R. 2003. "Dale's Cone of Experiences." http://teacherworld.com/potdale.html. Accessed June 24, 2012.
Phillips, L. 1987. "Closure: The Fine Art of Making Learning Stick." *Instructor* 97 (3): 36–38. http://www.eric.ed.gov. Accessed June 24, 2012.
Restak, Richard. 2006. *The Naked Brain*. New York: Harmony Books.
Wolf, P., and V. Supon. 1994. *Winning through Student Participation in Lesson Closure*. Distributed by ERIC Clearinghouse. http://www.eric.ed.gov. Accessed June 24, 2012.

Chapter 4

Reflections

FOCUS OF THE CHAPTER

In order for students to self-check their work and self-regulate their learning, they must be able to engage in reflection. Strategies and rubrics are available to helping student engage in the reflective process.

INTRODUCTION

As you read this chapter, ask yourself the following questions: What is the value of reflection? How is reflection used in lesson design? As you answer these questions think about how you and help your students self-check and self-modulate their work based on their reflection.

Probing Questions

1. What is the purpose of reflection?
2. Why is reflection necessary to empower teachers?
3. How can a teacher promote reflection for student self-regulation?
4. Why is reflection necessary to empower students?

WHAT IS REFLECTION, AND HOW DOES IT RELATE TO TEACHERS AND STUDENTS IN THE CLASSROOM?

Reflection—what comes to your mind when you hear the word reflection? If you are like most people, you think of a mirror and how you observe yourself at that moment. When you look into the mirror, either you decide that everything is just fine or you might decide to make changes to yourself.

You will use your reflection to give serious thought and consideration to what you see and decide what to do next. As educators we want to promote the same action of looking at something, making an assessment then planning a course of action.

This process is for the teacher to use in their lesson planning and during the instructional delivery and for the student to use to self-regulate their learning.

REFLECTION AS A TEACHER AND REFLECTION AS A SPORTS COACH

Let's start with reflection as it pertains to the lesson. For educators, the first thing that comes to their mind is a teacher reflecting upon his or her lesson to determine what went well and what needs to be revised. The revision is to improve the lesson so it will be more effective in delivery and subsequently lead to student achievement. Reflection is not only limited to teachers but also done by coaches and students.

For a sports coach, reflection usually occurs at the end of the game. At this time, the coach will determine what could have been done differently during the game, to improve the actions of the players.

For students, reflection can be done at the end of a lesson or during home learning time similar to what a sports coach would do. In both cases, reflection involves introspection of what had been done and what can be done differently. Introspection can be defined as the self-observation and reporting of conscious inner thoughts, desires, and sensations.

The process involves purposively relying on thinking, reasoning, and examining one's own thoughts, feelings, and actions. In education, this process is suggested to all teachers as a way to improve their instruction.

WHY REFLECTION IS IMPORTANT

This chapter will reveal why reflection is an important component of teaching, how reflection is strategically used by the teacher, and how to employ it on the student level.

REFLECTION TESTIMONY

Self-reflection allows a professional to think about where they are at that particular moment, in their career and assess their practice. The teacher who is complacent and content should reconsider how they can improve their craft. As a teacher, who has been through more than seven years of teaching English at primary and lower secondary levels, I have found myself in a position of a certain stagnation. At that phase, I started to ask myself more often; what [kind of] a teacher am I? To answer the question, I tried to look at my teaching from three different points of view." (Christodoulou 2010, 6)

TEACHER REFLECTION: BACKGROUND

Self-reflection is an important process for teachers. It creates an opportunity for them to think about what was done or what could be done. Reflection, when used with the proper "self" questioning techniques and personal insight, ensures that the teacher will delve into the lesson from another perspective.

A short scenario may help you better understand this point. Consider the teacher who has just completed a lesson or may be midway in a lesson with students. She believes that early on, that the lesson was going well, but she begins to see her students yawning, chatting, and not as focused. It is cause of concern for her. She stops and does a quick personal evaluation of her teaching methods and then makes an adjustment to the lesson.

Teacher's Dilemma

Many teachers are faced with the dilemma of continuing the lesson since time is their enemy and they need to get so much content completed, or to monitor and adjust the lesson which "takes away time from the lesson." What should that teacher do when she hits that bump in the lesson?

1. Should she continue, without reflecting on how the lesson's effectiveness is progressing?
2. If the teacher does reflect, she would need to assess what would be the reaction of the students once she does that mini midway evaluation of herself? Will the midway evaluation promote immediate changes within the classroom?
3. Does the teacher lose the opportunity to *discipline* "disruptive" students (the students not paying attention and seeking attention in other ways) by changing the lesson? (Are the students to blame for an ineffective lesson?)
4. Is the problem with the students or with the lesson construction?
5. How will self-reflection be used?

Possible Outcomes

One outcome to this scenario may be that there would be no change in the classroom atmosphere because the lesson was poorly planned and the teacher continues the lesson as she did not meet the student's needs.

Or, another outcome is that there was an *immediate change* in the classroom after the teacher reflected and adjusted the lesson. The critical aspect is that this teacher used *reflection* during her lesson.

Reflection after the Lesson

A critical point of reflection is that the teacher take more time after the lesson, to reflect upon their own teaching so they can plan more effectively for the next lesson. This teacher needs to examine what she actually did during the lesson, then come to a decision about what needs to be changed, in order to better prepare the lesson for the next time she teaches it. When the teacher steps outside the box and reflects upon her accomplishments she has grown not only professionally but personally as well.

This teacher is making professional and personal connections with her students that build a successful foundation for everyone. In order for educators to continually improve in the profession, it is necessary that they reflect upon their own teaching practice and ask deeper questions of what can be done differently, what worked, and what can be done to improve. It is this type of teacher reflection that is essential because it leads to consistent and constant improvement.

The Concept of Reflection

The concept of reflection is not new. Dewey (1933) believed that reflection is a process, for one to use to frame his or her way of thinking, so as to consider the current situation and propose ways of responding to future problems. Future problems can emerge from various contexts, including educational, social, and political. Reflection is also framed into shaping the environment.

In his text "Experience and Education," Dewey wrote that the primary responsibility of educators is that they must shape the actual experiences for the learner as well as recognizing what surroundings are conducive for having future experiences that lead to growth.

"Above all, they should know how to utilize the surroundings, both physical and social that exist, so as to extract all that they have to contribute to building up experiences that are worthwhile" (1933, 40). In essence, the teacher who had a problem with her class in the aforementioned example would reflect on the lesson and design an environment that is purposeful and promotes the establishment of student "sense and meaning" so the students see the value in what they are learning and regulate and modulate their learning in an environment that promotes self-regulation.

Reflection as Part of a Teacher's Evaluation

Many educators have developed rubrics for teacher reflection including Charlotte Danielson. Her rubric has four domains, and her domain 4 is titled "Professional Responsibilities." Danielson states, for that domain, "Teacher makes a thoughtful and accurate assessment of a lessons effectiveness and the extent to which it achieved, its instructional outcome, citing many specific examples from the lesson and weighing the relative strengths of each" (Danielson 2007, 94).

It is the highly competent teacher who reflects and understands what is necessary in the lesson, who is rated under Danielson's domain as distinguished or highly effective, while the teacher who does not know whether a lesson was effective or has achieved its instructional outcome is rated as unsatisfactory. In all cases, teacher reflection is important as it helps the teachers to perfect their craft. Professional growth is dynamic and not static.

Reflection Points

What are reflection points for a lesson? There are three particular types during a lesson. As educators we can reflect before, during, or after the lesson. Reflection "before" involves assessing student data and assessing data from a previous lesson to plan for a subsequent lesson.

Reflection "during" involves making mental notes throughout the lesson to determine if the lesson is effective. The reflection takes self-discipline as teachers often are eager to complete the lesson so their pacing becomes brisk. Reflection "after" occurs after the lesson. Please refer to Figure 4.1 for a schema of the reflection cycle.

Reflection After

Reflection after involves "going to the balcony" to look back and assess the lesson effectiveness. Both reflection "during" and reflection "after" are essentially reactive in nature, being distinguished primarily by *when* reflection takes place. As noted in Figure 4.1, Reflection After occurs after Consolidation for Closure.

Reflection During

Reflection "during" refers to reflection in the midst of practice and reflection "after" refers to reflection that takes place after an event. Reflection "before" begins the process of planning. Please refer to Figure 4.1.

In order for a teacher to be reflective during, the teacher needs to receive feedback from the students during the lesson he or she is teaching. The teacher should think through what is happening, and with the information he

78 Chapter 4

or she is receiving from the students, he or she can reshape the lesson without stopping. He or she will determine if what he or she is doing is effective and is understood by his or her students.

Based on the information that is received, the teacher can monitor and adjust his or her lesson. The monitoring and adjusting of the lesson can be called "temperature taking." Consequently, the teacher will be checking student outcomes frequently throughout the lesson, and he or she will use his or her feedback to *reflect* on whether he or she should reteach the concept or continue on with his or her lesson.

Based on the reflection in action, the teacher will monitor and adjust the lesson accordingly. It is the flow of interactive feedback that keeps the lesson fluid and meaningful to the student, as the teacher is making adjustments. This skill is a difficult skill as the lesson is usually planned.

Basically it would look like:

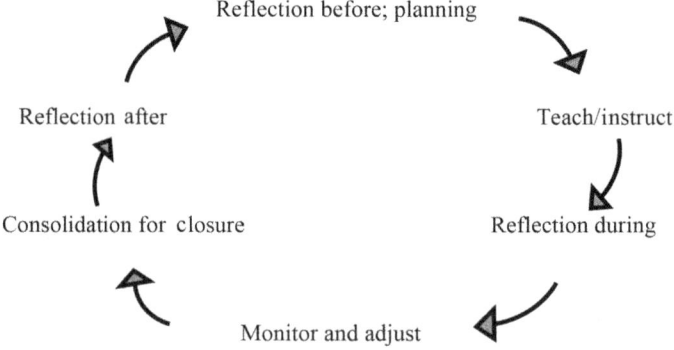

Figure 4.1

TEACHER REFLECTION

> Reflective thinking is always more or less troublesome because it involves overcoming the inertia that inclines one to accept suggestions at their face value; it involves willingness to endure a condition of mental unrest and disturbance. Reflective thinking, in short, means judgment suspended during further inquiry; and suspense is likely to be somewhat painful; to maintain the state of doubt and to carry on systematic and protracted inquiry—these are the essentials of thinking. (Dewey 1910, 13)

As stated earlier, teacher reflection is a key part of teacher growth and should become a practice in every teacher's career. It is the process of reflection, which will be the key to fine-tune a teacher's career.

A former teacher and college professor friend who spent a lot of time preparing for and delivering lessons shared an experience she had. Regarding the importance of reflection. After teaching a class on educational finance, she went home and told her husband that it was a great class and the students really enjoyed it. She told him that she taught the class about property tax and its relationship to a school budgets. He asked: How do you know they got it? How did she know? she replied: "I was there." "No, really, how do you know?" he asked again. This is when she began to think more deeply about the question. She told her husband that she instructs her students to keep daily journal. She collected their journals during each class and read them. It is through these journals that she sees what they learned from the lesson.

To her great surprise, many students reflected upon the lesson and expressed confusion about the process of determining property tax. Furthermore, they did not understand the formula to compute property tax. It was a lesson well learned for her.

From the student feedback, she learned: (1) it is important to do a Consolidation for Closure for each lesson in order to see what the students have retained and what they will reflect upon when they are out of class; (2) reflection is a powerful strategy for teachers as well as students, and more importantly, the follow-up from the reflection.

What Are Reasons Given for Not Doing Reflection?

When discussing reflection, teachers may state that reflecting is inconvenient, that they do not have time, or that they may feel it is not important to look over what they've done during the lesson. They may not see the value of using student responses in the "Reflection During" phase, so data are not interpreted when it is collected. Unfortunately, without reflection, teachers may never fully understand what information was actually learned by the student.

Teacher Evaluations Now Include Reflection

As part of the teacher evaluation, many school districts are now using the process of reflection. Reflection is an important component in the professional life of all teachers. Kim Marshall has developed a Teacher Evaluation Rubric (revised November 23, 2012). His model for observation in Section D—Monitoring, Assessment, and Follow-Up has ten indicators. One of the sections is reflection.

The assessment scale ranges from "Highly Effective (4)" to "Does Not Meet Standards (1)." The rating of highly effective (4) "works with colleagues to reflect on what worked and what didn't and continuously improve instruction." A rating of "Effective (3)" is "reflects on the effectiveness of lessons and units and continuously works to improve them." A rating of "Improvement Necessary (2)" "at the end of a teaching unit or semester, thinks about what might have been done better." A rating of "Does Not Meet Standards (1)" "does not draw lessons for the future when teaching is unsuccessful."

Marshall is gracious in allowing the use of the rubrics, as he states that the rubrics are "open source" and may be used and adapted by schools and districts as they see fit.

Danielson also has a rubric for assessing teachers, and it consists of four domains. Domain 4 is "Professional Responsibilities." The section on reflection assesses the teacher's thinking, which follows any instructional event, so that the teacher can analyze the many decisions made in the planning and implementation of a lesson.

Danielson incorporated this component, since its importance has an impact on student learning. Teachers can determine where to focus their efforts when making revisions, and what aspects of the instruction they will continue in future lessons. Teachers may reflect on their practice through collegial conversations, which can be part of a Professional Learning Community (PLC) or by the Critical Friends process.

THE PROCESS OF REFLECTION

Teacher must learn, as well as practice, the process of reflection. The reflection process begins with an accurate assessment of what was done, and then formulation of a plan on how to proceed, after the lesson is analyzed for future teaching. Although reflection is a learned skill, it can be developed and tweaked with other teachers present, with mentors, coaches, and supervisors.

The professionals will begin by asking the proper probing questions. Over time, this way of thinking and analyzing instruction, through the lens of student learning, becomes a habit of mind. An administrator may ask a teacher to submit lesson plans/assignments/unit plans from multiple years that show change/growth/adaptation in order for that teacher to learn how to reflect on his or her own teaching.

Learning from Our Experience

Experience can be an effective teacher as long as it doesn't kill one in the process. So, the adage that we learn from our experience is true but more accurately, we learn from the reflection that comes after our action. It is the metacognition that is important and the use of reflection to refine our thinking.

American teachers would do well to reflect more on the details of their time spent with students. American schools, and administrators, would do well to foster this professional development by providing time, support, and varied structures, in which the exercises can be carried out.

Lesson Study

In Japan, it is common practice for elementary and middle-school teachers to collaboratively develop, execute, reflect upon, and refine individual lessons. This professional practice is most often referred to as "lesson study," but more accurately it is lesson research. It provides teachers a formal framework through which they engage in careful reflection, about their students' learning.

The product of a Japanese lesson study is not only the refined lesson, but also the greater benefit that comes to each teacher, from time spent engaged, with colleagues, in deep and meaningful reflection of his or her practice. An important aspect of this exercise is its focus on *the lesson*, not on the performance of individual teacher(s), who delivers the information, during the lesson study.

The focus of the conversation is always the lesson and its aspects, not whether an individual teacher taught well or not. This distinction, though it may seem insignificant, is cited as critical, in setting the tone for this professional activity. Teachers are engaged in seeking best practices, as a team, rather than critiquing one another.

Teacher Reflection or with a Little Help from a Friend

Most teacher evaluation systems (Danielson, Marshall, Marzano, and others) encourage teachers to reflect on observed lessons. They may even encourage teachers to discuss their reflections with the observer, presumably a supervisor or principal. In order for benefit to be derived from this conversation, however, two conditions must be satisfied.

First, the observer must be a competent teacher and evaluator, knowledgeable in pedagogy and content and able to communicate her observations based on research and not opinion. Second, the climate of the school, and the tone of this specific interaction, must be non-threatening enough, so that the teacher can self-assess honestly and engage in open dialogue about strengths, weaknesses, and goals.

Given these conditions, the best model, for promoting teacher reflection, is to divorce it from teacher evaluation, and structure it as professional learning. When and if teacher's salaries become tied to performance evaluations, it will be more important that teachers engage in reflection toward genuine professional improvement. Allowing teachers to work with colleagues on coaching walks, peer walkthroughs, or to engage in action research (e.g., through PLC lesson study) would be a much more effective model for promoting teacher reflection and teacher improvement.

Reflection Is Not a New Concept—Ask John Dewey

The notion of reflection is not a new concept, but one that was proposed by John Dewey. It is the heart of intellectual organization and of the disciplined mind (Dewey 1938). John Dewey saw reflection as a rigorous way of thinking. When reflection occurs, it must also happen within our attitudes and school community as well.

Reflective practice yields several primary benefits for teaching. Professionals become more confident and skilled through this practice. There are numerous instances where teachers used previous notes to revise approaches to a particular concept, broader topic, or assignment and observed that the revision led to increased student comprehension in the next class.

It is crucial for teachers to regularly question, reflect upon, and improve their teaching practices. Currently in New Jersey, districts are moving toward evaluation systems that will implement and enhance each teacher's reflection process. All teachers can develop habits of mind conducive to effective decision-making.

Reflection is a skill which also can be fostered with colleagues. Coworkers who demonstrate expertise in posing and solving problems often prove to be good mentors. These persons are adept at their skill and are able to listen analytically enabling them to focus on key information that helps clarify and direct the teachers into this new deeper thinking model.

Another way to help teachers become better at reflection is to create study groups that introduce teachers to different modes of thinking. Discussions and role-playing can help teachers see which routine decisions can be made through technological or situational thinking and which may require the deliberate or dialectical modes. Identifying different types of thinking modes appropriately assists teachers to use their time and mental energies wisely.

Reflection on practice may be constructed differently for everyone, but in all cases it means constructive criticism, being honest to oneself, and becoming aware of and understanding one's own feelings. Teachers have to affirm: "I want to make sure that I am the best teacher that I can be. All of my students should gain something from having me as an effective teacher, so I should be willing to hone my craft so as to teach in an effective way."

If teachers are not currently performing at mastery level or near it, then they should reflect on their current practices and learn to enhance their skills and techniques. The climate of education is constantly changing, and teachers must reflect upon their own practice, in order to stay current on best practices, and meet the needs of their students. What may have worked in the classroom years ago may not be relevant today. What may work for one student may not work for another. These ideas should guide teacher reflection and growth.

Teacher Empowerment

Teachers are aware of their actions and consequences, remain willing to change, and maintain the belief that all students can learn. In order for teachers to truly be reflective, they seek and embrace opportunities to learn. Teacher empowerment begins with a cyclical process of inquiry, reflection, and application of the concepts for growth. Just as we encourage our students to become lifelong learners, teaching requires a willingness to learn and grow professionally.

Taking Control of One's Life

If teachers are reflective, they will be empowered to do well, which is the key to more effective teaching. By taking control of their teaching lives, they become empowered decision makers who can then begin to act on their world in a way that can change it.

Reflective practitioners come to see themselves as change agents capable of knowing the present and creating the future. Sometimes teachers may feel that there is nothing they can do to improve a situation; they feel powerless. This type of thinking, which blames the students or the circumstances, is dangerous and leads to complacency.

Through reflection, teachers have an opportunity to influence their practice much more than they may think! Reflection encourages the teacher to be an "action researcher" and not "passive consumer." By examining an area of concern and actively seeking out a solution, it empowers teachers because they can make a change in their own classrooms, which will immediately impact the learning of their students.

Just as educators encourage meaningful learning experiences for their students through self-regulation, teachers will also be more likely to improve if they feel a part of the process. The only person who can change a teacher is the teacher!

Reflection Can Be a Group Activity

Although we typically think of reflection as a solitary process, sometimes the involvement of others leads to more meaningful reflection. An environment that promotes *collaboration,* *cooperation,* and *dialogue* leads to greater learning among teachers. For example, if an educator has an area of concern, he or she can request a peer to observe that particular area and ask for feedback.

Another way for group reflection is for a teacher to discuss issues in a PLC meeting and through collaboration discover a different strategy from colleague input.

If a collaborative, reflective environment is encouraged in a school, other teachers can be a valuable resource. In a similar sense, an administrator can also help a teacher become more effective by being a facilitator in the teacher's professional growth. By involving the teacher in the process of evaluation and asking for teacher feedback, in a post-observation conference, the administrator and teacher can work together to create a strategy for continued development.

Rather than, "this is what I see you are doing right and/or wrong," comments from the administrator, a reflective approach involves the teacher as an integral part of his or her own growth and development as a professional and master teacher.

Reflection and Professional Development

In addition, reflective practice leads to more effective professional development. In a traditional model of professional development, strategies are provided to educators but may not be based on the teacher's personal need. The assumption is that the professional development provided will lead to behavioral change and better performance in the classroom. However, there is little evidence that this approach works well, especially if the teacher does not see or feel the need for professional development. They lack a growth mind-set.

Lacking a perceived need, teachers return to the classroom and fall back into the same routine. Change does not stem from standard information suggested by an expert in a large group. Rather, true change comes from self-awareness. When the teachers evaluate their own practice and come to their own conclusions, their practice will improve. Just as we are encouraged to differentiate instruction for students, administrators need to ensure that the teachers see the need or have the need for professional development.

Professional development should be directed at the areas teachers need to improve. For example, if student engagement is a concern for some teachers, they would specifically benefit from professional development in that area. If professional development is not designed in this way, it becomes a missed opportunity for enhancing classroom instruction.

Teacher reflection has great value, and teachers can request specific professional development based on their reflection. Teacher reflection should be highly regarded by all teachers and administrators. It is critical for a district to promote a reflective community that empowers the teachers and provides them with the support necessary to make changes. It is only by creating this environment through collaboration and professional development that true change will occur and teacher effectiveness will improve.

Teacher Reflection and Lesson Development

Each day a teacher must assess students, make quick decisions, and account for meeting their daily objectives and responsibilities. Teaching the curriculum is a small portion of the day.

Teacher reflection is a vital component to effective teaching. Initially, when creating a lesson, the teacher must continually be mindful of what, why, and how he or she is planning.

Lessons must be relevant, creative, and planned at a student's instructional level. Next, at the conclusion of each lesson, the teacher must consider the following: student engagement, attention, participation, relevance, progress, and performance, to name just a few of the key components to evaluate the lesson. These are just some of the factors to review when determining if the lesson was successful or not.

Upon completion of this review, the next lesson must be tailored to meet the needs of the class, as per the Core Curriculum Content Standards. An additional way to reflect upon one's methodology is to review assessment results.

For example, given twelve students in a class, if a quiz is given and eight students earn Ds, two earn Cs, and two earn Fs, then clearly the students do not understand the concept. As a result, the teacher must consider the possibility that the lesson was ineffective or the assessment was unfair. Once he or she determines this, then he or she needs to determine why to further explore the lesson.

Additionally, classroom management, seating, and environment are other areas of teaching that must be reflected upon to ensure a positive learning climate for our students. The reflective process must be an ongoing component of educational planning.

STUDENT REFLECTIONS

Why Is Reflective Thinking Important?

It is increasingly important to prompt reflective thinking during learning to help learners develop strategies to apply new knowledge to the complex situation in their day-to-day activities.

The role of reflection on planning is critical. Reflection provides insight and learning from experience. Done consistently, reflection benefits the entire learning community. Reflection is a way students can understand their own experiences and translate them into understanding their unique strengths and challenges. Reflection additionally compels students to give careful consideration and ask questions about learning styles, multiple intelligences, brain research, and gender-based differences. Reflection before, during, and after the lesson teaching provides information to produce growth.

Students should maintain reflective journals in writing/language arts areas. Both students and teachers can examine work samples to gain insight into what, why, and how the reflective process is working. The teachers will review, make comments, converse with students, conduct student/teacher conferences, or simply ask the students to think about their own style of learning, while they think about their own style of teaching.

Reflection helps students by asking key questions of themselves and share their information with teachers who will begin to learn what connections students are making or what they need to make for their students in order to build successes.

Questions to Promote Student Self-Reflection

A natural way of promoting student self-assessment and reflection is through asking questions such as the following:

1. What do I really understand about x?
2. Why did it make sense to me?
3. What is still confusing you?
4. What do I need to do to get information to clarify my confusion?
5. How can I improve?
6. Will I use the rubric provided to assess where I am and what I have to do to improve? I will self-regulate my learning using rubrics.
7. If I did not do as well as I thought, what would you I differently next time?
8. What were the strengths I exhibited?
9. Why do you think you did well and how can it be applied to future learning?
10. What were my deficiencies in _____? What will I do differently next time, including how I studied?
11. How does your preferred learning style influence how you learn, and will you use a different learning style to study for the next assignment?
12. Why does what you learned make sense?
13. How can you apply what you learned?

STUDENT REFLECTION: SRL PRACTICES

The True Level of Understanding Is Evident in the Kinds of Questions Students Ask Teachers

Teachers, who model open-ended questioning techniques, stimulate student reflection. Open-ended questions also generate the students' need to know more information thus beginning the process for student self-regulation. The use of open-ended questions helps begin the process of introspection and metacognition.

The process of student self-monitoring begins with student action; however, the teacher should model how the student can begin the process. The teacher can ask the student to reflect on the following questions as a prompt to student self-regulation.

1. Is the result you achieved what you had expected to achieve?
2. Are you satisfied with the outcomes?
3. If the outcome was not what you expected, what will you do differently?
4. Will there be other resources or aids you can use to gain the desired result?
5. Did you monitor your progress along the way or wait until the end?
6. Was that an effective strategy? Why or why not?

Research to support self-management was a study by Mooney et al. (2005), who reviewed literature from the past to 2005. This review reported on the effectiveness and focus of academic self-management interventions for children and adolescents with emotional and behavioral disorders.

Twenty-two studies published in twenty articles and involving seventy-eight participants met inclusionary criteria. The overall mean effect size (ES) across those studies was 1.80 (range: 0.46 to 3.00), indicating effects were generally large in magnitude and educationally meaningful.

Self-monitoring interventions were the predominant type of self-management technique used by researchers. The mean ES for intervention types were self-evaluation (1.13), self-monitoring (1.90), strategy instruction techniques (1.75), self-instruction techniques (2.71), and multiple-component interventions (2.11). Interventions targeted improvement in math calculation skills more than any other area. The mean ES by academic area were math interventions (1.97), writing (1.13), reading (2.28), and social studies (2.66).

Refocusing the lenses through reflection will, and does, promote teacher and student growth and deeper learning.

The next chapter will provide sample lesson plans applying what has been discussed.

BIBLIOGRAPHY

Christodoulou, Iva. 2010. *Teacher Self-Reflection: Diploma Thesis*. Masaryk University, Faculty of Education, Department of English Language and Literature. BRNO, 6. https://is.muni.cz/th/266245/pedf_m/DPIva_Christodoulou.pdf.
Creasap, Sally A., April L. Peters, and Cynthia L. Uline. 2005. "The Effects of Guided Reflection on Educational Leadership Practice: Mentoring and Portfolio

Writing as Means to Transformative Learning for Early-Career Principals." *Journal of School Leadership* 15 (4): 352–86.

Danielson, Charlotte. 2006. *Teacher Leadership That Strengthens Professional Practice*. Alexandria, VA: Association for Supervision and Curriculum Development.

———. 2007. *Enhancing Professional Practice: A Framework for Teaching*, 2nd ed. Alexandria, VA: ASCD.

———. 2008. *The Handbook for Enhancing Professional Practice: Using the Framework for Teaching in Your School*. Alexandria, VA: Association for Supervision and Curriculum Development.

Dewey, John. 1910. *How We Think*. Boston, MA: Heath.

———. 1916. *Democracy and Education*. New York: Free Press.

———. 1933. *How We Think: A Restatement of the Relation of Reflective Thinking to the Educative Process*. Chicago, IL: Henry Regnery and Company.

———. 1938. *Experience and Education*. New York: Collier Books.

Fosnot, Catherine. 1989. *Enquiring Teachers, Enquiring Learners: A Constructivist Approach to Teaching*. New York: Teachers College Press.

Garner, Betty K. 2007. *Getting to "Got It!": Helping Struggling Students Learn How to Learn*. Alexandria, VA: Association for Supervision and Curriculum Development.

Grant, C. A., and K. M. Zeichner. 1984. "On Becoming a Reflective Teacher." In *Preparing for Reflective Teaching*, ed. C. A. Grant, 103–14. Boston, MA: Allyn & Bacon.

Jackson, Anthony. 2013. "Japanese Lesson Study." *Global Learning*. Education Week, January 4, 2012.

Killion, Joellen P., and Guy R. Todnem. March 1991. "A Process for Personal Theory Building." *Educational Leadership* 48 (6): 14–16.

Mooney, Paul, Ryan, Joseph B., Uhing, Brad M., Reid, Robert, and Epstein, Michael H. Sep 2005. "Review of Self-Management Interventions Targeting Academic Outcomes for Students with Emotional and Behavioral Disorders." *Journal of Behavioral Education* 14 (3): 203–221.

Tomlinson, Carol Ann, and Jay Mctighe. 2006. *Integrating Differentiated Instruction and Understanding by Design: Connecting Content and Kids*. Alexandria, VA: Association for Supervision and Curriculum Development.

Wideman, Jim. August 17, 2012. *5 Key Self-Reflections for Leadership Growth*. http://www.churchleaders.com/pastors/pastor-articles/162310-5-key-self-reflections-for-leadership-growth.html.

Yoshida, Makoto, and Clea Fernandez. 2012. "Overview of Lesson Study in Japan." globaledresources.com. rbs.org (Research for Better Schools). Accessed June 20, 2013.

Chapter 5

Sample Lesson Plans
Putting It All Together

In order provide an example of how the Learner's Brain Model can be applied in a lesson, attached is a sample lesson plan that incorporates the Learner's Brain Model. Although the comments are specific to this lesson, they can be applied to any other lesson. As you review this lesson, look at the comments under each section, and think: How can this comment apply to my lesson.

LESSON PLANNING

Teacher: Christine Casale
Lesson: Create an Advertisement
Unit Topic: Persuasive Writing
Grade level: Sixth

Essential Questions

Why is persuasive writing important? How do we use persuasive writing in our own lives? How do we persuade others? How do persuasive messages influence us? What makes a good argument? Why is a writer's choice of words important? How do the rules of language affect communication? How do writers develop a well-written product?

Comment: The Essential Question is consistent with the brain's processing of visual information in a holistic manner. In essence, the brain is looking for a pattern in which the visual—"visual thinking"—is connected to the end goal. Basically, the brain is looking to determine if there is a pattern in which a relationship to what is being taught is evident. We know this fact when we are all shown an optical illusion. We look to see a pattern but the illusion causes the visual impression to be compromised. Like an optical illusion, the brain must sort out the new stimuli (the lesson) with what they already know. The Essential Question is the beginning of the pre-delivery (readiness stage) of the Learner's Brain Model. Once the student know the Essential Question, (big picture, end goal), the Student Learning targets (objectives) make more sense as they are the short term goals which will help to achieve the big picture.

Student Learning Target (Objective: Written Student-Friendly)

I will be able to apply and evaluate persuasive strategies as well as use persuasive writing skills through oral discussion.

Comment: Set objectives which are student friendly as the objective is for the student and not for the administrator. Throughout the lesson provide feedback to the students to focus the on the objective. This is important as this begins the process of self-regulation on the student's part. Most importantly, it is necessary to use prompts or gestures to refer back to the objectives and the Essential Question to focus student attention and "forward frame" the information for future use.

Start and reinforce a lesson with questions and/or advance organizers.
The Learner's Brain Model on lesson design addresses the issue of starting a lesson by using a Readiness Set. It helps to bridge the new information to prior information so as to motivate and focus the student.

Student Learning Target (Objective)

Comment: An effective lesson will begin with the teacher ensuring that students are aware of the purpose and objectives of the lesson. Learning objectives of the lesson should be clearly posted on the board or wall and will be reviewed with the class. The classroom teacher should communicate what the students should expect to learn during the lesson, why it is important, and what the students will be doing to achieve these objectives; otherwise, the students are constantly searching for "meaning." If students understand the purpose and objectives of the lesson, it will help them assess themselves throughout the lesson to see if they are meeting the lesson objective so they are engaged in self-regulation. Do not set the instructional goals too specific as it may lead the student to focus too narrowly on the goal and ignore other relevant information not specifically related to the goal.

An effective objective ties in students' prior knowledge and connects to other parts of the students' curriculum and experiences. This will increase student engagement as the objective becomes more relevant and meaningful to the students.

Demonstration of Student Learning

Art Smart/Visual-Spatial

I will create an advertisement and commercial using the writing process and receive at least a 3-point on a 4-point rubric.

Verbal-Linguistic Students

I will also show the teacher that I mastered the skill by completing a peer/self-assessments and evaluation form and by sharing my results with the teacher in a teacher/student conference.

I will be able to review persuasive strategies and identify strategies used in a passage and on Post-its, creating an advertisement and commercial using the writing process.

Interpersonal

I will be completing peer/self-assessments and evaluation forms, sharing work, and participating in teacher/student conferences.

Comment: Lessons require daily DSLs by all students as it measures the attainment of objectives. Additionally, the information obtained from the DSL will be useful for planning Differentiated Instruction. Keep in mind that the DSL is only one form of formative assessment, so using DSLs and checks for understanding, the teacher will be able to gain valuable information to monitor and adjust the instruction.

STANDARDS TO BE ADDRESSED

Comment: Use standards-based planning so students will know what the expectation level is that they are being held accountable to achieve. The standards will also allow feedback to be given to the student based on established expectations and norms. All lessons should be planned using standards.

The use of standards will also help to bring focus on the teacher's planning and consistency to all teachers if all teachers across grade levels use them to plan. A problem would occur if some teachers were using one set of standards, that is,

Common Core Curriculum Standards (CCCS) or Common Core State Standards (CCSS), while other teachers were using state standards that are different from the Common Core State Standards. Some standards may be covered at different grade levels so the curriculum would not be articulated.

Writing

- CCSS.ELA-Literacy.W.6.1: Write arguments to support claims with clear reasons and relevant evidence.
  - CCSS.ELA-Literacy.W.6.1a: Introduce claim(s) and organize the reasons and evidence clearly.
  - CCSS.ELA-Literacy.W.6.1b: Support claim(s) with clear reasons and relevant evidence, using credible sources and demonstrating an understanding of the topic or text.
  - CCSS.ELA-Literacy.W.6.1c: Use words, phrases, and clauses to clarify the relationships among claim(s) and reasons.
  - CCSS.ELA-Literacy.W.6.1d: Establish and maintain a formal style.
  - CCSS.ELA-Literacy.W.6.1e: Provide a concluding statement or section that follows from the argument presented.
- CCSS.ELA-Literacy.W.6.4: Produce clear and coherent writing in which the development, organization, and style are appropriate to task, purpose, and audience.
- CCSS.ELA-Literacy.W.6.5: With some guidance and support from peers and adults, develop and strengthen writing as needed by planning, revising, editing, rewriting, or trying a new approach.
- CCSS.ELA-Literacy.W.6.6: Use technology, including the Internet, to produce and publish writing as well as to interact and collaborate with others; demonstrate sufficient command of keyboarding skills to type a minimum of three pages in a single sitting.

Comprehension and Collaboration

- CCSS.ELA-Literacy.SL.6.1: Engage effectively in a range of collaborative discussions (one on one, in groups, and teacher-led) with diverse partners on grade six topics, texts, and issues, building on others' ideas and expressing their own clearly.
  - CCSS.ELA-Literacy.SL.6.1b: Follow rules for collegial discussions, set specific goals and deadlines, and define individual roles as needed.
  - CCSS.ELA-Literacy.SL.6.1c: Pose and respond to specific questions with elaboration and detail by making comments that contribute to the topic, text, or issue under discussion.

- CCSS.ELA-Literacy.SL.6.3: Delineate a speaker's argument and specific claims, distinguishing claims that are supported by reasons and evidence from claims that are not.

Presentation of Knowledge and Ideas

- CCSS.ELA-Literacy.SL.6.4: Present claims and findings, sequencing ideas logically and using pertinent descriptions, facts, and details to accentuate main ideas or themes; use appropriate eye contact, adequate volume, and clear pronunciation.
- CCSS.ELA-Literacy.SL.6.6: Adapt speech to a variety of contexts and tasks, demonstrating command of formal English when indicated or appropriate. (See grade six Language standards 1 and 3 here, for specific expectations.)

Conventions of Standard English

- CCSS.ELA-Literacy.L.6.1: Demonstrate command of the conventions of standard English grammar and usage when writing or speaking.
- CCSS.ELA-Literacy.L.6.2: Demonstrate command of the conventions of standard English capitalization, punctuation, and spelling when writing.

Knowledge of Language

- CCSS.ELA-Literacy.L.6.3: Use knowledge of language and its conventions when writing, speaking, reading, or listening.

  - CCSS.ELA-Literacy.L.6.3a: Vary sentence patterns for meaning, reader/listener interest, and style.
  - CCSS.ELA-Literacy.L.6.3b: Maintain consistency in style and tone.

Vocabulary Acquisition and Use

- CCSS.ELA-Literacy.L.6.6: Acquire and use accurately grade-appropriate general academic and domain-specific words and phrases; gather vocabulary knowledge when considering a word or phrase important to comprehension or expression.

READINESS SET

The Learner's Brain Model uses a Readiness Set to get the students' interest at the onset of a lesson or at the beginning of a new lesson. After the

Readiness Set, the teacher plans the lesson to "make sense" and have meaning for the students. This phase is stage 1 of the Readiness Cycle.

The emphasis on setting the stage for learning fits precisely with the current research on the attentional mechanisms of the brain. Our brain immediately starts sifting and sorting through all the sensory input. At the same time, the brain searches through previously stored information and looks for relevant hooks for the new information. A Readiness Set increases the possibility that the brain will search through the right networks and attend to the information that is relevant for a particular topic or issue.

Examine the advertisement on the Smart Board. In your Do Now Journals, answer the following questions: What are they trying to sell? What persuasive strategies do they use? Are they successful? Students will share their responses with a partner, and the class will discuss the effectiveness of the advertisement as well as the strategies used.

Comment: The cognitive principle is that your "memory is not a product of what you remember, is a product of what you think about" (Willingham 2010, 43). The students need to see the relationship of what they are learning so the material becomes relevant. To help achieve this concept, a Readiness Set is used to hook the students' interest, connect the students' prior knowledge, and tie both to the lesson so the lesson will make sense and have meaning.

The concept of Readiness Set is to focus student attention. The process is a way to help students organize and think about the content, see a direct link with what they previously studied, or help the students recall what they already know.

INSTRUCTIONAL INPUT

This lesson will be part of a unit on persuasive writing. By this point, students will have been exposed to persuasive strategies such as testimonial and bandwagon.

Comment: The critical variable is that the teacher would have assessed their students to know where their students are and can plan appropriately. (More detail about Instructional Input is in Chapter 2.) Once the students are appropriately assessed, the teacher can tier the lesson based on student needs.

The purpose of the lesson is for the students to not only develop their persuasive writing skills but also apply these skills in a real-world context.

Comment: This is critical for authentic learning as students need to know what they are learning has an application. If students do not see the application, the usual question is: "Why do we have to know this?" or the real killer question: "Will this be on the test?" If the teacher answers no, the student will fail to see the value of the information and may "shut down."

Students will review the persuasive strategies learned by discussing their graphic organizer as well as identifying and evaluating strategies in sample advertisements around the room. After the review of the strategies, students will be responsible for creating their own advertisements and commercials in groups. The advertisement must use the persuasive strategies the class learned. It must include an illustration, slogan, and reasons to purchase the product or service. Students will also create a commercial where they must sell their product or service. They should create a jingle for the commercial. The advertisement and commercial must also include price comparisons and environmental implications of the product or service.

Comment: The use of creativity is important as the students get to apply what they are learning in a new way.

If we teach for competency, we may not get performance. Students will know how to do a problem but lack the skill to apply it. If we teach for performance where the students have to show what they know, we automatically get competency. The Learner's Brain Model stresses metacognition via application so students develop competency and apply what they know.

Visual

A sample advertisement will be displayed on the Smart Board during the Do Now. Persuasive strategies with examples will be presented in a graphic organizer for easy reference. Sample advertisements will be posted around the room. Models, assignment rubric, and the assignment sheet will be shared with students and displayed on the Smart Board.

Comment: Using model and visual representations is stressed in math instruction and is one of the new shifts for the Common Core. The Learner's Brain Model stresses on establishing the physical environment, developing emotional security, mood, and climate as important for the classroom domain and establishing an environment conducive to learning. Establishing a classroom environment that has safety, emotions, novelty, humor, music, choices, physical movement, hands-on activities can contribute to increased alertness and memory. When a varied approach is used, the information is processed by the brain via the various modalities, i.e., visual information is processed in the visual part of the brain.

Auditory

Students will share their Do Now findings with a partner in a Think-Pair-Share activity. The class will discuss the Do Now findings as a large group as well. The teacher will review the persuasive strategies through oral discussion when referencing the graphic organizer. After reviewing the handout, students will be asked to share with a partner at least three strategies that they think are most effective. The class will also review the sample advertisements together after students label them with Post-it notes. The teacher will review the models, rubrics, and assignment sheets orally asking students questions and providing students with the opportunity to also ask questions.

Upon completion of the entire project, students will share with the class. As groups are presenting the advertisement and commercial, the rest of the class will complete an evaluation form noting the persuasive strategies used. As a large group, the class will discuss their findings and the effectiveness of the advertisements and commercials.

Research has also shown that while threats impede learning, positive emotional experiences, during which the brain produces certain chemicals or neurotransmittersand does promote learning. Negative experiences inhibit learning. I would contend that all learning is "emotional" in that positive experiences promotes learning.

Comment: Research has shown that the brain's limbic system, located just above the brain stem at the base of the brain, is responsible for our emotional responses. Neuroscientists have determined that new information that comes to the brain is processed first in the emotional center before being processed in the cognitive center, located in the frontal lobe of the cerebrum. With information processing short-circuited first to the emotional center, chronic stress may impair long-term memory and learning. The effects of stress and learning have significant implications for educators and hence the Learner's Brain Model stresses establishing a safe emotional environment for students so they can participate in class discussion, debates, or critiques of their peers work or presentation.

Tactile

Students will respond to the Do Now by writing in their journals. To review persuasive strategies, students will be shown various sample advertisements. They must be able to write the persuasive strategy used in the sample advertisements on a Post-it note.

Kinesthetic

Students will then have to place their Post-it note under the correct advertisement.

Concrete Sequential

Rubric and assignment sheet will be provided to present tasks in an organized manner. Rubrics are used as checklists to self-regulate. Models and sample advertisements will be shown and can be referenced freely throughout the class. The teacher will conference with the students to ensure that expectations are clear. Students are making original products because they are creating an advertisement. They also are creating graphs and charts for the price comparisons. Creating the advertisement and commercial is a hands-on activity to a practical problem that requires realistic writing.

Abstract Sequential

Models and sample advertisements will be shown. Part of the assignment requires an illustration. Research of prices and environmental implications is also necessary. The project requires problems-solving skills and synthesis to convey one clear advertising goal based on reason. The element of argument is present because students are constructing persuasive advertisements to convince others to purchase their product or service. There is also individualized study because each group member has specific tasks to accomplish. Lecture is used when the project is introduced. Outlining and note-taking will also be used in the brainstorming stage.

Concrete Random

Students will be working in small groups. There is an aspect of problem-solving and use of real-world experience in the lesson because they need to determine how to market their product. Students are creating an advertisement and commercial, which require innovation and divergent thinking as well as a hands-on experience. Brainstorming and gathering information is needed before creating the final product.

Comment: Use real materials such as familiar tangible objects to demonstrate concepts and make ideas more concrete. For example, when teaching about ice, water, and steam, use real-life objects to teach the concepts.

Use chants and rhymes while learning, as rhythmic patterns stick to the brain.

Movement and humor are also important. Dance, sign, play games, and laugh as these activities will use multiple sense and will increase memory.

Abstract Random

Students will be working in small groups on varying tasks with benchmarks for completion. Models of the project will be shared. Teacher feedback is provided to all students throughout the entire project. Illustration is part of the requirement for the advertisement and role-playing is required in the commercial. There is also an element of music necessary in the commercial for the jingle. Creative writing is also needed for both the commercial and advertisement.

MODELING

The teacher will review the persuasive strategies presented on the graphic organizer. The teacher will then reference the sample advertisements around the room. Students must determine which strategies are used in the advertisements and if they are effective. The teacher will model how to determine the persuasive strategies used in the first advertisement. After students review the persuasive strategies, the teacher will review the rubric and assignment sheet for the advertisement and commercial with the students, so expectations are clear. The class will be presented with several models and a rubric that can be referenced freely throughout the class. Students will have an opportunity to ask questions.

Comment: During this time, the instructor will share with the class a time they have received help from an unlikely source. The instructor will help the students understand that sometimes you may receive help without even realizing it. The instructor will help the students prepare for the lesson through this discussion by scaffolding into the story for the class. The teacher will tie in help from a source to using self help or self regulated strategies to achieve a goal.

INPUT (ACTIVITIES)

Students will share with a partner three persuasive strategies that they find most effective. The teacher will then ask the students to examine the sample advertisements around the room and on a Post-it note write the strategy they think is being used. Students will be asked to place their Post-it note under the advertisement.

After review of the first activity, the students will be divided into randomly selected groups, where each student will be assigned specific tasks to complete. Each group will receive a card with a product or service like cereal or bakery. However, they are able to make the product or service their own by creating its own brand, including a name and identifying features. Students must complete their brainstorming and rough drafts prior to completing the final project. Students will use a rubric throughout the project for self-assessment purposes. They will complete a group assessment rubric at the end of the lesson to ensure that all students are accountable for contributing to the group.

Comment: The more senses involved during learning, the more likely the brain will receive and process information. By using multiple senses to learn, children find it easier to match new information to their existing knowledge.

The brain research is very clear, the brain performs many functions simultaneously. Learning is enhanced by a rich environment with a variety of stimuli.

Hands-on activities increase sensory input, which helps learners attend better.

Present content in a variety of teaching strategies such as physical activities, individual and group instruction, and artistic and musical variations helps orchestrate student experiences.

GUIDED PRACTICE

The teacher will circulate and monitor progress when the students are recording the strategy on the Post-it notes.

Comment: After the teacher feels comfortable with the progress of the lesson, keeping in mind the notion of primacy-recency, there may be a point in the lesson for students to do independent practice. The teacher must monitor the student's progress to ensure that the student has the knowledge and appropriate skills to do the activity independently. As the teacher monitor's the student progress she must keep detailed notes and must have enough feedback to ensure that the student has the knowledge and appropriate skill to do the activity independently. The research done by Marzano, Pickering, and Pollock revealed that mastering a skill requires focused practice and even suggests that it's not until students have practiced "upwards of about 24 times that they reach 80 percent competency" (Marzano, Pickering, and Pollock 2001, 67).

Once in groups for creating the advertisement and commercial, the teacher will monitor progress and circulate among groups to make sure that students are staying on task and answer any questions. Students must first brainstorm using a graphic organizer. As the students complete their brainstorming and rough drafts, they will be shown to the teacher before creating the final project. The teacher and student will discuss strengths and areas in need of improvement.

CHECK FOR UNDERSTANDING

To ensure that the students understand the strategies before moving onto the group part of the project, the teacher will review the identified strategies that the students wrote on the Post-it notes and students will discuss the effectiveness. Teacher will also encourage students to ask questions after discussion of the project so expectations are clear.

Once in groups, teacher will check brainstorming and rough drafts of each group prior to creating the final product. Teacher will chunk activities and give estimated completion times. Groups will provide the teacher with status updates of their projects. Students will share their graphic organizer with a partner and be encouraged to ask their group questions for clarification throughout the project. Students will use a rubric to self-assess and peer-editing throughout the project to self-regulate and ensure that they are on task. Once the project is completed, students will also present their projects, complete evaluation forms, and engage in large-group discussion about the effectiveness of the advertisements/commercials.

Comments: During the activity, there will be frequent checks for understanding using a variety of strategies. The instructor will see if the children have understood what was being said and if their answers are accurate by sharing their answers with the class. During this time, the students will be chosen randomly to help get all the students involved in the discussion and to make sure the children are participating. Participation is not an option. At this time the class will construct a KWL chart based upon the answers sheets. This chart will help to show what the class already knows, learned, and what they want to learn in this lesson. The KWL chart will show the teacher what the class will be held in the front of the class and will be added to as the information is learned or to add anything new that the students may want to learn. This chart will be an ongoing process in this lesson.

Teacher can also use other ways to check for understanding—visual, tactile, or kinesthetic.

MULTIPLE INTELLIGENCES

Linguistic

Students will use their persuasive writing skills to create the advertisement and commercial. Students must consider their target audience. They must brainstorm convincing reasons to purchase their product or service as well as what differentiates their product or service from competitors. They must also create a slogan. Specific persuasive strategies must be used.

Logical–Mathematical

The students must show the price of their product or service in comparison to other competitors using graphs and charts in their advertisement and commercial. (Students will use the internet to research prices so they can make accurate comparisons.)

Musical

Students will create a commercial to sell their product or service using persuasive strategies. As part of the commercial, students can add a jingle.

Bodily Kinesthetic

Students will create a commercial to sell the product or service. They will have to physically act out the commercial. Students will need to move freely around the room to work with others and gather supplies for each task.

Spatial–Visual

Students will be asked to create an illustration as part of the advertisement. The picture should support the persuasive strategies used.

Interpersonal

Students will be working collaboratively in groups throughout the entire project. Students must be able to ask questions of their peers and share progress. Work must be divided; however, through collaboration, it must all communicate the same persuasive goal. The students will keep a journal of their findings.

Intrapersonal

Each student within the group will have certain tasks to accomplish independently. They will keep a log of their tasks and self assess their progress.

Naturalist

Students are encouraged to make their product/service environmentally friendly, so they must examine the environmental implications of their project. (Computers may be used to research environmental impact of product or service.)

LESSON PLAN

Teacher: Ms. Smith
Focus: Author's Purpose
Grade: Second

Objective

I will be able to identify the author's purpose and justify my reasoning.

Demonstration of Student Learning

I will correctly identify three important element of the story and provide supporting evidence for my choices.

Read Aloud: "Schools around the World"
Cross-Content Connection: Social Studies
Standards: RF2.3f, RF2.4c, SL 2.1a, L2.6

OPENING/MINI-LESSON

Brief Vocabulary Review

Prior to the beginning of the lesson, a five-minute review on key vocabulary is done. Reteach strategies on decoding and word analysis for vocabulary words. These are words that are present in the story and will increase vocabulary development.

Diverse: Things or people that are different from each other
Literacy: The ability to read and write

Resources: Materials, money, and other things that can be used
Culture: A group's customs or traditions
Uniform: Clothes that all of the people in a group wear so they are dressed alike
Proper: The way it is supposed to be; correct

Display pictures of schools and classrooms from different countries on the board. Open the discussion by triggering the students' memory.

Comment: The review of the vocabulary will get student attention and make it meaningful.

Ask the children to discuss some memories from their school experience. After a few selections, refer to the pictures of different schools. Allow students to note details in the picture by comparing and contrasting their lives and the pictures.

Comment: Brain research says that the frontal lobe is processing information when students talk. Talking and walking promotes metacognition. Having students talk about their memories makes the information personal and meaningful.

Comment: The Readiness Set in this lesson involves a think-pair-share activity that is extremely important because brain research has found that learning is emotional and that permanent learning almost always has an emotional component. Memory and learning are closely tied to emotions. Having the students interact with one another works best because it gets the students interested and engaged in their own learning. In addition, the brain remembers information more readily when it is meaningful and can be linked to prior knowledge or experience.

On the gathering area, display a KWL graphic organizer on a chart. Discuss with the children that they are going to read a book about schools around the world. Filling in the chart together, ask students questions for each section of the KWL chart. "What do you know? What do you want to know? And afterward, what have you learned." Each section will be color-coded for easy reference.

Comment: Brain research explains that using color increases learning by promoting visual imprinting.

Inform the students that the Essential Question is related to the author's purpose. "What is the purpose of the selection?" "Why did the author write this story?" Call on two students to make a prediction about the story. (Begin reading the story.)

Comment: Throughout the story, stop and ask questions about the literature. This will give the students the opportunity to engage in critical thinking, hypothesize, predict, visualize, evaluate, and draw conclusions. As discussed in the text, prediction has value in promoting retention.

Prediction is also a great tool for increasing comprehension. After the story, we will summarize and discuss important details from the story.

Comments: Address all levels of Bloom's taxonomy—literal, inferential, and creative levels. It is suggested that teachers continue to effectively engage students in meaningful ways and differentiate instruction based on students' readiness and academic needs. Essential Questions written in lesson plans and posted in classrooms will assist the teachers in developing more rigorous questioning types. Thoughtful lesson planning that targets higher-order thinking skills enables students to "get the big picture" and transfer learned knowledge to new and different situations.

In order for students to be actively engaged in learning, the students need to be mentally involved in understanding the lesson content and are participating and contributing to the instructional lesson. Teacher needs to be asking cognitively challenging questions that will ensure that the students are thinking. Questions should have more than one answer and should not be simple "yes" or "no" questions. Research indicates that questions that require students to use higher-level thinking skills produce more learning than questions that require student to recall or recognize information. It is important to allow "wait" time after posing a question as this will allow a greater depth of student responses. In addition, all classroom activities and assignments should require students to think broadly and deeply, problem solve, and engage in critical thinking.

WORK PERIOD

Distribute a number to each child from one to four. There will be four traveling stations in the classroom. The number will determine the students' placement. At each station, there will be a question related to the story and four minutes for each member to answer. Students will discuss opinions and experiences regarding the lesson. After four minutes, the timer will go off, and each group will move to the next station. Once the groups are at their starting point, students will return to their seats for independent work. Students will complete a Venn diagram comparing and contrasting our school and the schools in the story.

Comment: Hands-on activities increase sensory input, which helps learners attend better. Questions posed at each station will be used to focus student attention and to ensure that they are "on track." Otherwise students will go to a station and discuss anything or talk about topics not related to the assignment.

Centers

Comment: The brain is always seeking the big picture—the pattern of thought that is created by repeated use of familiar neural pathways.

Listening Center: Listen to "Schools around the World." Students can listen to the same story on tape. Those students having difficulty with comprehension or low-leveled readers can use the audio and picture book for assistance.
Writing Center: Students will write five facts about their school. They will also draw a picture to go with their sentences.
Technology Center: Kidbiz, Learning.com, or Starfall.
Free-Time Center (Sensory Enrichment): Students will have a variety of materials and resources to explore and stimulate conversations with each other. This center allows for discovery and explanation from areas such as foods, geography, family, community, senses.
Guided Reading: Focus: Author's Purpose. Read the story "What We Do in Schools." Use this story to connect it to the read aloud from the opening lesson. This is also an opportunity for increased personal connections.

CLOSING MEETING

The students will reconvene in the gathering area. We will restate our objective and discuss the story again. Some students will be called upon to share their Venn diagram. Teacher will also call upon one person from each center to discuss what they did and how it connected to today's lesson. The students will complete our KWL chart. Teacher will also ask students questions regarding the story to informally check for understanding.

Comment: The nature of classroom talk is complicated and too little understood. While there is evidence that more "thoughtful" classroom talk leads to improved reading comprehension (Fall et al. 2000; Johnston et al. 2001; Nystrand 1997), especially in high-poverty schools (Knapp 1995), we still have few interventions available that focus on helping teachers develop the instructional expertise to create such classrooms and few of the packaged programs offer teachers any support along this line. True conversation cannot be scripted or packaged. The classroom talk observed should be highly personalized and focused on a targeted reply to student responses. Teacher expertise is the key and not a scripted, teacher-proof, instructional product.

Below is an example of how to incorporate the Differentiated Instruction (DI) rubric for grade two Everyday Math Lesson Data Day by Mrs. Dorothy Lusk. Mrs. Lusk is the general education teacher in the grade two inclusion classroom at William J. McGinn Elementary School in Scotch Plains, New Jersey. She has been teaching fourteen years in the primary classroom including kindergarten, first, and second grades. Mrs. Lusk incorporates her special educational background into the regular educational classroom in order to meet the needs of the varied learners from students who receive both support and pull-out services to very bright and highly motivated students. Differentiation occurs both through varying academic difficulty and varying modalities of learning in order to provide many ways for students to access instruction at a level that is both developmentally appropriate and interest engaging.

DIFFERENTIATED INSTRUCTION

The following lesson is from grade two, Everyday Math. I have taught the lesson in the past using the procedures from steps 1 to 8; step 9 has been created and added to this lesson to follow Differentiated Instruction Activities. Additionally, I adapted the Differentiated Instruction Chart, page 2, copyrighted by Dr. Mario Barbiere, to be used as a tool to check on the effectiveness of this specific lesson and its components. The chart could be used to check any lesson for Differentiated Instruction. Each of the lessons' tasks and activities is aligned according to the standards of a rubric from highly effective to ineffective. The rubric assesses student engagement in the areas of content, process, product, interest, and readiness "look-fors."

Comment: The rubrics can be used for preplanning a lesson, during a lesson, or reflection after a lesson.

Sample Lesson Plans 107

MATH: LESSON 6.3 DATA

CCCS: 2.MD.5, 2.MD.10
Vocabulary: Basic food groups, Food Guide Pyramid, data table, bar graph

Objectives

1. I will demonstrate the ability to collect, sort, tally, and graph data.
2. I will demonstrate the ability to locate and identify food items in the food groups using a grocery store circular as a connection to real life.
3. I will be introduced to the concept of science and nutrition as it is connected to everyday math and real life.
4. I will demonstrate an understanding of the reality of limited spending within a budget.
5. I will demonstrate the ability to create a daily menu to reflect an understanding of a balanced diet and without and within budgetary restrictions.

Procedures

1. The teacher will display a model of the former version of the Five Basic Food Groups on the ELMO as the guidelines for second graders: Lead a discussion regarding how the food groups work and what each part means, including the fact that although there are five basic food groups.

   Comment: The more senses involved during learning, the more likely the brain will receive and process information. By using multiple senses to learn, children find it easier to match new information to their existing knowledge. In addition to a multi-sensory approach, having student talk is an effective strategy.

2. The teacher will guide the students in a shared reading activity in which each student views his or her own math journal page depicting the new U.S. Department of Agriculture model of Food Groups. Each group will work together on the task: Compare the two models and create a list of what you notice to share with the class—you should notice both similarities and differences. Allow the students to notice that the pyramid is divided into six parts because the U.S. Department of Agriculture divided up the fruits/vegetables and added a category for fats/sweets (TE 391).

   Comments: Brain research supports that lifelong learning best occurs when students are able to apply content, skills, and processes to tasks that require them to engage in higher-order thinking and problem-solving skills. Using knowledge meaningfully requires students to extend thinking by examining concepts in deeper, analytical ways, thus requiring the brain to use multiple and complex systems of retrieval and integration. Modules from one part of the brain connect to other modules when we perform complex tasks. Problem-solving activities that include cognitive components such as memory, language, emotion, and active learning engage the motor cortex.

Limit the number of new concepts taught per day. For example, when teaching first grader about food groups, begin with only one food group at a time.

Summarizing and note-taking reduces the amount of information the learner needs to get into long-term storage. Each is a form of a chunking strategy.

Children are better able to focus on important information when they receive less, rather than more, information.

When you reduce the amount of information to be learned, there is a better chance for it to be stored in the long-term storage.

3. The teacher will tell the class that as part of their study of Food Groups they will be choosing various activities to learn about the Food Groups and how they fit in everyday life.

    Comment: Classroom rituals and specific opening and closing routines provide beginning and endings of class segments and also add an emotional component for a safe environment. Kids like routines as the routines help with class management. Additionally, have routines and expectations informs.

4. The teacher will display grocery store circulars and pose the question: "Have you ever seen one of these? What is it? What could we use it for? How does it help a consumer?"

    Comment: The Readiness Set also helps to establish a readiness for what will be coming and to establish a safe emotional environment.

    The anticipatory set in this lesson involves a think-pair-share activity that is extremely important because brain research has found that learning is emotional and that permanent learning almost always has an emotional component. Memory and learning are closely tied to emotions. Having the students interact with one another works best because it gets the students interested and engaged in their own learning. In addition, the brain remembers information more readily when it is meaningful and can be linked to prior knowledge or experience.

5. The teacher will allow the students to peruse the circulars briefly. He or she will have the students discuss what they notice about the circulars with

Table 5.1. Lesson activity Distribution

	Anchor activities	Choice board (#9)
Whole Class	Introduction (#1) Display and distribute circulars (#5)	• Create a life-sized Food Pyramid on class bulletin board—students take turns cutting items out of their circulars and placing them in the correct category of the Food Pyramid.
Individual	Shared Reading Food Pyramid (#2) Favorite Meal (#7)	• Use the circulars to locate prices for favorite food in order to make the meal. • Write Journals: Do you think making healthy food choices is important? Explain why or why not.
Partner	Ingredients of favorite meal (#8)	• Create graphs based on Tally Chart of Favorite Food Ingredients for Food Pyramid. • Graph choices. • **Low:** Picture or bar graph with assistance to determine setup of graph. • **Middle:** Bar graph agreed-upon set up by the partners with mode and range identified. • **High:** Pie graph with percentages/fractions identified and marked. • Use the menu costs to determine change from a given dollar amount possible amounts: $20, $50, $100.
Small Group	Compare Food Pyramids (#3) Peruse circulars/compare circulars (#6)	• Tally Chart of Favorite Food Ingredients for Food Pyramid Categories. • Set up menu for the day with balanced food choices. • Use the menu and circulars to estimate a realistic cost of the menu. • Complete a balanced menu within a budget. • Analyze the cost of each category of the pyramid: Is one category more expensive than another?

The following table has been adapted from Differentiated Instruction Table.
Copyrighted by M. Barbiere, Ed.D. April 2013, September 2013.

their table groups and quickly share out their "noticing" including: format, location of items by category, pictures, prices, and varieties of product—name brands/store brands. He or she will tell the students that they will be using the circulars at some of the choice board activities. The task is to engage the students emotionally in the lesson.

Comment: Emotions drive attention and attention drives learning and memory. Things become real to the brain when we feel them emotionally. Emotions affect memory and brain functions. Jensen (2005) notes

Table 5.2. Rubric for Differentiation of Instruction

Dispositions—"look fors"	Highly effective student engagement	Highly effective considerations or tasks	Specific math lesson objectives/procedures/activities highly effective
Content **"Look fors"** Standards-based, interdisciplinary, rigorous, student-centered, authentic	• Whole group lesson leads to individual, partner, and small-group activities. • Teacher-directed and student-selected activities. • The teacher will guide the students in a shared reading activity in which each student views his or her own math journal page depicting the new U.S. Dept. of Agriculture model of Food Groups	• Interdisciplinary lesson with high level of application. • Problem-based learning demonstrates deeper understandings. Each group will work together on the task: Compare the two models and create a list of what you notice to share with the class—you should notice both similarities and differences. Allow the students to notice that the pyramid is divided into six parts because the U.S. Dept. of Agriculture divided up the fruits/vegetables and added a category for fats/sweets (TE 391) understanding	Interdisciplinary Lesson—Math/Science/Social Skills/Health. Whole Group: (see above chart) Individual: (see above chart) Partner: (see above chart) Small Group: (see above chart) Teacher-Directed: Introduction to Lesson—Food tables Student-Selected: Choice Boxes Problem-based Learning Activity: Food Choices, Costs, Graphing The grouping of students into high, middle, and low will allow for student interest, student readiness, and student product to be factored into the lesson for differentiation.
Process **"Look fors"** Structured, dynamic, monitored and adjusted based on feedback; promotes SRL	• Students move at their own pace and self-manage their time. • Student selects activities in addition to anchor activity.	• Centers set up with materials needed. • Students work with partner or small group and manage their time to complete the activity. • Choice board is posted to choose activity—mandatory activity is in place for all to manage.	Time schedule is posted to complete each activity and each student has his or her own folder to manage materials when time is called. Anchor Activity: Center and choice boards to determine each Student-Selected Activity Multiple Intelligences Visual/Spatial: Use of circulars, Food Pyramids, graphs, and tally charts.

	• Flexible grouping is used to group students. • Students use multiple intelligences	*Bodily/Kinesthetic:* Awareness of proper diet, moving around to various centers. *Logical/Mathematical:* Calculate the cost of food items and determine how to fit within a given budget. *Verbal/Linguistic:* Use of written and oral language to complete various charts and graphs and explain results or findings. *Intrapersonal:* Metacognition thinking about what is best for healthy diets and determining which food group a choice belongs to and identifying own food choices—ability to balance healthy and unhealthy lifestyles. *Interpersonal:* Working with a partner or small group cooperatively.
Product **"Look fors"** **Summative, diverse, Multiple Intelligence (MI) used, shows what student know, understand, or do**	• Real-world application. • Use MI to create product based on student ability. • Information is analyzed, interpreted, and created. • Activities demonstrate what each student knows and understands or can do independently and in a small group or partnership.	• Use circulars to make food menu choices for a balanced meal. • Use circulars to estimate costs and compute real costs within a budget. • Multiple Intelligences: Student-selected choices encompass various learning styles as outlined in above table box. • Food choices are analyzed for nutritional balance and cost. • Menus are created according to given criteria.

(Continued)

Table 5.2 (Continued)

Dispositions— "look fors"	Highly effective student engagement	Highly effective considerations or tasks	Specific math lesson objectives/procedures/ activities highly effective
Interest "Look fors" Student involvement activities, student connections, self-regulation	• Specific references to students' interests are highlighted throughout the activities. • Real-world student connection is made. • Students self-regulate their choices.	• Tasks involve real-world procedures and expectations for daily living. • Students identify their own choices and complete the assignments based on personal choice not on one-size-fits-all choice.	Students choose foods according to own likes and preferences. *Real-world connections* *Healthy diets lead to long lives.* *Living within a budget.* *Favorite foods are used as a hook to generate interest.*
Readiness "Look fors" Student skill levels, grouping, assessments to determine levels	• Pre-assessments are made to determine grouping. • Teacher assistance/ resources are available for students with special needs in order to have same level of choice as typical peers. • Writing Journals: Do you think making healthy food choices is important? Explain why or why not it is an example of promotion of self-regulation. The teacher will review student journal to determine what feedback can be given to promote self-regulation.	• Each specific task has more than one level of difficulty, depending on the task. • Final products based on MI. Using MI is one way to provide a way of understanding intelligence, which teachers can use as a guide for developing classroom activities that address multiple ways of learning and knowing. Teaching strategies informed by MI theory transfer control from teacher to learners by giving students choices in the ways they will learn and demonstrate their learning.	Food Pyramid on ELMO compared/contrasted with New Guidelines Pyramid. Grouping for graphing based on previous graphing activities outside of this activity. Making change amount is also based on previous estimating and making change activities outside of this activity. In class, support teacher is available to assist with or modify activities as needed in addition to predetermined groupings. Some activities are leveled within the task. Final products based on MI.

that when a person feels content, the brain releases endorphins that enhance memory skills.

6. Before separating the group, the teacher will ask every student to write down his or her favorite meal. "display your own favorite meal (For example, pizza, salad, and Diet Coke)."
7. Tell the students they will be working with their partner to list the ingredients that are used to make up their favorite meal. (dough-bread/grains, mozzarella cheese—dairy, tomato sauce—vegetables, salad—vegetables, dressing-fats/oils, Diet Coke—no food value). Once this is done these will be collected for use of one of the choice board activities.
8. The students will be divided into groups/partners with various tasks from the choice board assigned to differentiate this lesson. Hands-on manipulation increases the chance by 75 percent that new information will be stored in long-term memory (Hannaford 1995; Sousa 2006). Hands-on activities increase sensory input which helps learners attend better.

LESSON ACTIVITY DISTRIBUTION

After my own analysis of how to differentiate the lesson, I realize how much more student-directed the learning becomes with a relatively small amount of teacher-directed instruction to enable the students to complete many tasks that include a real-world application and meaning. Regardless of what evaluation model a district uses, New Jersey teachers are being evaluated based of the rigor of the lesson, the quality of questioning involved, the real-world application of the student activities, the actual knowing and understanding of the product, the ability of the students to self-regulate their learning in a meaningful manner, and the assessment of the learning in order to generate future lessons, and ways to best instruct the students. Interdisciplinary instruction is also becoming the only way to fit the increasing demands of a vast and demanding curriculum.

As for our students, Differentiated Instruction enables all students to learn to their highest potential by virtue of the use of multiple intelligences and a variety of tasks designed to meet all learners' needs not a one-size-fits-all model. Differentiated Instruction takes practice and requires a commitment; however, productive learning leads to application far beyond simply that lesson and the application is what truly demonstrates understanding and the acquisition of useful knowledge.

BIBLIOGRAPHY

Anderson, L.W., Krathwohl, D.R., Airasian, P.W., Cruikshank, K.A., Mayer, R.E., Pintrich, P.R., Raths, J., Wittrock, M.C. 2001. *A Taxonomy for Learning, Teaching, and Assessing: A revision of Bloom's Taxonomy of Educational Objectives.* New York: Pearson, Allyn & Bacon.

Bloom, B. S. 1954. University of Chicago. Churchill, Ruth. Antioch College. Cronbach, L. J. University of Illinois. Dahnke, Harold L., Jr. Michigan State University. Detchen. . . . J. French, Accent on Teaching. New York: Harper & Bros., 1954.

———. 1956. *Taxonomy of educational objectives: The classification of educational goals handbook I: Cognitive domain.* New York: David McKay Company

Caine, R. N., and G. Caine. October 1990. "Understanding a Brain-Based Approach to Learning and Teaching." *Educational Leadership* 48 (2): 66–70.

Dalton, J. and Smith, D. 1986. "Extending Children's Special Abilities – Strategies for primary classrooms" pp. 36–7. http://www.teachers.ash.org.au/researchskills/dalton.htm

Danielson, Charlotte. 2007. *Enhancing Professional Practice: A Framework for Teaching*, 2nd edition. Alexandria, VA: Association for Supervision and Curriculum Development.

Elder, Janet. "Findings about Brain Research and Brain-Friendly Instructional Strategies." www.readingprof.com.

Fall, R., Webb, N. M., and Chudowsky, N. 2000. "Group discussion and large-scale language arts assessment: Effects on students' comprehension." *American Educational Research Journal* 37: 911–941.

Hannaford, C. 1995. *Smart moves: Why learning is not all in your head.* Arlington, VA: Great Ocean Publishers.

Hardiman, Mariale. 2012. *The Brain Targeted Teaching Model.* Baltimore, MD: Johns Hopkins University Press.

Hunter, M. 1979, October. "Teaching Is Decision Making." *Educational Leadership* 37 (1): 62–67.

———. 1982. *Mastery Teaching.* El Segundo, CA: TIP Publications.

Jensen, Eric. 2005. Teaching with the Brain in Mind by Eric Jensen – Applying brain research in your school system. Association for Supervision & Curriculum Development, VA.

Johnston, P., Woodside-Jiron, H., and Day, J. 2001. "Teaching and learning literate epistemologies." *Journal of Educational Psychology* 93: 223–233.

Knapp, M. S. 1995. *Teaching for meaning in high-poverty classrooms.* New York: Teachers College Press.

Kuzmich, L. (2011) in Anderson, L.W., Krathwohl, D.R., Airasian, P.W., Cruikshank, K.A., Mayer, R.E., Pintrich, P.R., Raths, J., Wittrock, M.C. 2001. *A Taxonomy for Learning, Teaching, and Assessing: A revision of Bloom's Taxonomy of Educational Objectives.* New York: Pearson, Allyn & Bacon.

Marzano, R. J. 2007. *The Art and Science of Teaching: A Comprehensive Framework for Effective Instruction.* Alexandria, VA: Association for Supervision and Curriculum Development.

Marzano, R. J., D. Pickering, and J. E. Pollock. 2001. *Classroom Instruction That Works: Research-Based Strategies for Increasing Student Achievement*. Alexandria, VA: Association for Supervision and Curriculum Development.

Marzano, Robert. 2006. *Classroom Assessment and Grading That Work*. Alexandria, VA: Association for Supervision and Curriculum Development.

Nystrand, M. 1997. *Opening dialogue: Understanding the dynamics of language and learning in the English classroom*. New York: Teachers College Press.

Schiller, Pam, and Clarissa A. Willis. July 2008. "Using Brain-Based Teaching Strategies to Create Supportive Early Childhood Environments That Address Learning Standards." *Young Children* 63 (4): 52–55.

Sousa, David. 2000. *How the Brain Learns*. Thousand Oaks, CA: Corwin Press.

———. 2001a. *How the Brain Learns*, 2nd edition. Thousand Oaks, CA: Corwin Press.

———. 2001b. *How the Special Needs Brain Learns*. Thousand Oaks, CA: Corwin Press.

———. (2006) *How the Brain Learns*.

Stape, Chris. September 28, 2009. "Brain Research, Instructional Strategies, and E-Learning: Making the Connection." *Learning Solutions Magazine*. Retrieved from: learningsolutionsmag.com.

Willingham, D. T. 2010. *Why Don't Students Like School?*, in *Why Don't Students Like School?: A Cognitive Scientist Answers Questions About How the Mind Works and What It Means for the Classroom*. Jossey-Bass, San Francisco, CA, USA.

Wolfe, Pat. 1999. Revisiting Effective Teaching - Educational Leadership – ASCD www.ascd.org/publications/educational.../nov98/.../Revisiting-Effective-Teaching.asp. November 1998, Volume 56, Number 3, pp. 61–64.

Appendix A
Rubric 1: Questioning

Knowledge Dimension	Factual Knowledge Basic Elements to Know	Conceptual Comprehension	Procedural: How to Do an Analysis Evaluation	Metacognition Create
Create	Assemble, elaborate	Generate, produce, propose	Design, devise, how would you test . . .	Create, compose, improve
Evaluate	Judge, appraise, deduce	Predict, critique, prioritize, argue	Justify, verify, debate, evaluate	Reflect, rationalize, prove
Analyze	Infer, distinguish compare, contrast	Compose, organize, categorize, analyze	Illustrate, cause/effect, differentiate	Deconstruct, attribute, make a chart
Apply	Show, explain, build, organize	Solve, produce	Extend, apply, generalize, solve	Use, implement
Understand	Demonstrate, explain, give examples, match, paraphrase	Classify, interpret, distinguish	Recognize, show, summarize	Conclude
Remember	Recall, match, choose, find, label, name	Locate info, recall, recite, show, find	Describe	Identify from a list
	Teacher-Directed			Student-Directed

Source: Bloom (1954 and 1956) revised by Anderson and Krathwohl (2001), examples from Dalton and Smith (1986) and Kuzmich (2011).

Teacher Activity: Lecture, Review, and so on	Revised Bloom's Taxonomy (RBT) Category	Verbs	Instructional Strategies	Model questions
	Remember	Choose, describe, find, identify, label, list, name, recall, recite, recognize	Highlight, memorize, make a list, make a chart	Who? Where? What? How? When? What does it mean?
	Understand	Demonstrate, distinguish explain, give examples, match, paraphrase, show, summarize	Students explain, state a rule, paraphrase, visual representation	Statement on words, What does it mean? Give an example, Explain what is happening, What is the main idea? Is this the same as . . .? What are they saying? What seems likely?
	Apply	Apply, explain, generalize, judge, organize, produce, show, sketch, solve, use	Apply in the real world, case study, construct a model, explain an idea	Predict what would happen, Tell me how, when, where, and why? Identify the results of . . .? What is the function of . . .? Choose the best statements that apply . . ..
	Analyze	Analyze, categorize, cause/effect compare, contrast, differentiate	Jigsaw activity, What are the assumptions and relationship?	Is that fact or opinion? What are the assumptions? What does the author believe? What is the relationship between..? State a point of view or pattern. What is the motive?
	Evaluate	Appraise, argue, estimate, criticize, debate, justify, verify	Justify, prioritize and rationalize, debate, evaluate	Invalid? Judge the effects, find errors, defend your point of view, justify your answer, isn't biased, fair, or ethical?

Teacher Activity: Lecture, Review, and so on	Revised Bloom's Taxonomy (RBT) Category	Verbs	Instructional Strategies	Model questions
	Create	Compose, construct, design, device predict	Design, create, devise, or compose	How would you test, develop creative solution, invent a new system, process, and procedure?

Source: © M. Barbiere., May 2012, February 2013, March 2013. Used with permission of the author.
Dr. Barbiere's text, Activating the Learner's Brain, 2018, Rowman and Littlefield, Lanham, MD.

Teacher: _____ **Room:** _____ **Grade:** _____ **Date:** ____

		Questioning	Indicators	Questions/Verbs
Highly Effective		- Questions are of high quality - Verbs are consistent with create level of revised Bloom's Taxonomy - Teacher allows adequate response time - Wait time is more than five seconds - Teacher questions help students formulate questions - Promote cognitive stimulation	- Questions promote cognitive stimulation and discussion, not recitation - Questions are divergent - Questions promote thinking and help students make connections - Questions are open-ended	What new product can you create? How would you test, develop creative solution, invent a new system, process, procedure? How would you test, develop creative solution, invent a new system, process, procedure? Compose, construct, design, device predict
Effective		- Many questions are of high quality - Verbs are consistent with evaluation level of revised Bloom's Taxonomy - Teacher is sporadic with regard to response time - Wait time is three to five seconds - Teacher questions help students formulate analytical type of questions Promote some cognitive stimulation but not rigorous	- Questions promote some cognitive stimulation and some questions are convergent - Teachers probe answers to questions - Questions cause students to evaluate information, no cognitive challenge or creation of new ideas - Questions allow for exploration of content	Valid or invalid? Judge the effects, finding errors, defend your point of view, justify your answer, isn't biased, fair, or ethical? Appraise, argue, estimate, criticize, debate, justify, verify, analyze, categorize, cause/effect compare, contrast, differentiate

Partially Effective	- Questions are a combination of low and high quality - Verbs are consistent with mid-level of revised Bloom's Taxonomy (apply and analyze) - Teacher allows adequate response time - Wait time is more than one to two seconds - Teacher questions help students comprehend material - Promote marginal cognitive stimulation	- Some Questions are narrow, convergent - Questions allow for some student reflection - Questions cause the student to analyze information, but still not cognitively challenging	Predict what would happen, tell me how, when, where, and why? Identify the results of.. ? What is the function of . . .? Choose the best statements that apply . . .. Apply, explain, generalize, judge, organize, produce, show, sketch, solve, use
Ineffective	- Questions are of poor quality and single correct responses - Verbs are consistent with low level of revised Bloom's Taxonomy - Teacher allows adequate response time - Wait time is less than one second - Teacher questions help students recall information - Promote limited cognitive stimulation	- Questions are narrow, convergent - Questions are rapid fire - Questions recall information, no cognitive challenge - Questions are yes/no	Demonstrate, distinguish explain, give examples, match, paraphrase, show, summarize, choose, describe, find, identify, label, list, name, recall, recite, recognize
Student Questions	- *How do the teacher's questions promote new understandings or better understand the content?* - *Does the teacher's questions promote thinking and help you see connections?*	- *Guiding Question: What are the students doing as a result of what the teacher has said or done?* - *Are the students cognitively challenged or compliant?* - *As a result of the teacher's questions, the student are challenged to arrive at new understanding*	

Source: © M. Barbiere, May 2012, March 2013. This rubric is copyrighted; permission to use must be obtained.

Dr. Barbiere's text, Activating the Learners Brain, 2018, Rowman and Littlefield, Lanham, MD.

Appendix B

Rubric 2: Student Engagement

Student Engagement

Teacher: _____ Room: _____ Grade: _____ Date: _____

	Student Engagement	Indicators
Highly Effective	- Activities are student-directed and planned for student involvement. - Students initiate or adapt activities or assignments - Materials and resources promote student engagement - Lesson has high degree of student involvement as teacher facilitates the lesson. - Multiple instructional strategies used. - A variety of learning styles are used in the delivery. Auditory, visual, and tactile experiences are provided. - Multiple responses strategies are employed - Student initiate choice, adaption, or creation of materials	- Students know what to do when they enter the room and begin to work independently - Cooperative activities are planned or group work is conducted. Teacher facilitates the process. - Multiple learning styles are used throughout the lesson. - Students are able to self-regulate their learning either by self-management or self-monitoring - Multiple response strategies used - Teacher checks of understanding every 5–7 minutes and adjusts accordingly.
Effective	- Activities vary from student-directed to teacher-directed. - A majority of time devoted to student involvement. - Materials and resources promote student engagement - Lesson has high degree of student involvement as teacher facilitates the lesson. - Multiple instructional strategies used. - A variety of learning styles are mostly used in the delivery. Auditory, visual, and tactile experiences are provided. - Multiple responses strategies are employed	- Students know what to do when they enter the room and begin to work independently - Cooperative activities are planned or group work is conducted. Teacher facilitates the process. - Multiple learning styles are addressed sporadically throughout the lesson. - Some students are able to self-regulate their learning either by self-management or self-monitoring - Multiple response strategies used sporadically. - Teacher checks of understanding every 8–10 minutes and adjusts accordingly.
Partially Effective	- Activities are appropriate to some students. - Materials and resources do not promote students for all students - Lesson has sporadic student involvement but more teacher-directed - There is marginal student involvement as most of the lesson is teacher-driven. - One learning style (auditory) is used during the lesson. - Limited multiple responses, mostly choral responses	- Some activities are varied for students - There is some student activity as students are working - Two learning styles are used but most of the instruction is lecture. - Some students will know what to do but most wait for the teacher to direct them. - Teacher checks for understanding and uses one or two strategies.
Ineffective	- Students come late; enter the room and wait for the teacher to tell them what to do. - Students are compliant but not intellectually engaged - Lesson is teacher-driven. - One learning style is used during the lesson (auditory) - Students not sure of what to do next, cannot regulate their own learning - No multiple responses strategies - Few checks for understanding	- Activities are teacher-directed with minimal student involvement. - Lecture-driven lesson with little student involvement. Students are compliant but not engaged. - Students need to be told what to do or will frequently ask the teacher what to do next. - Teacher has limited checking for understanding and continues lesson after a few students respond
Student Questions	- What are you expected to do when you enter the class? - What do you do if you finish early? - What are your responsibilities for group work	- Guiding Question: What are the students doing as a result of what the teacher has said or done? - Are the students cognitively challenged or compliant? - Can students manage and monitor their time effectively and independently?

© Copyright, M Barbiere, May 2012, March 2013. This rubric is copyrighted; permission to use must be obtained.
In Dr Barbiere's text: *Activating the Learner's Brain*, (2018), Rowman and Littlefield, Lanham, MD.

Student Engagement

Overall Rating: _____

Follow-up: ____ yes ____ no

Follow-up Date: _____

Notes:

_____
_____
_____
_____
_____
_____

Next Steps:

_____
_____
_____
_____

Student Engagement "Look Fors"

Learning styles used	
Multiple response strategies used	
Checking for understanding	
Self-monitoring or self-management	
Independent learner	
Teacher facilitation	

© Copyright, M Barbiere, May 2012, March 2013. This rubric is copyrighted; permission to use must be obtained.
In Dr Barbiere's text: *Activating the Learner's Brain*, (2018), Rowman and Littlefield, Lanham, MD.

Appendix C

Rubric 3: Student Interviews

Student Interviews

	What are you learning? (Forethought: Phase 1 of SRL, Wolter, 2010)	How do you assess your learning? Monitor Learning: Phase 2 Zimmermann, 2000)	Why studying? Use, management and regulation of learning strategies: Phase 3	When you need assistance? Reflection: Final stage of SRL
Highly Effective	- Student explains learning in specific and concrete terms. - Student provides an analysis of the learning. - Students are aware of the criteria for a specific project or task. - Student describes the expected outcome.	- Students use the learning environment (exemplars, rubrics, posted work) to assess their learning - Students monitor their learning - Conduct a similar DOL as the one by the teacher—adapting activities	- Student evaluates the lesson and makes a real world connection - Student demonstrates self-regulation strategies for the expansion of the lesson - Student relates the learning to goals (EQ or unit) and career	- Students identify others who can help them - Students seeks other sources for assistance - Students develop ways to self-regulate - Students develop and use ways to self-manage their time and work - SRL strategies used
Effective	- Student explains more than the lesson objective - Student explanation is clear and specific - Student makes connections to other disciplines - Student uses "I" statements" or indicates self-monitoring in another manner	- Teacher feedback used - Students are aware of the rubric for use to self-monitor or assess - Peer review used - Written feedback from assignments used to promote learning - Multiple ways used to assess student learning is a better sentence.	- Student able to make a connection to real world situations - Student can explain necessary milestones for the next grade or graduate - Student dispositions or habits of mind exhibited for higher level learning. - Student can apply the lesson to future learning	- Student knows three options before asking the teacher - Student frequently uses the classroom environment for assistance. - Student uses notes, work folders, journals to self-regulate the learning.
Partially Effective	- Student states the learning objective only. - Student restates objectives using "I".	- Limited use of assessments by students - Student has a source for assessing their learning, in the room or personally, but is not used.	- Student occasionally self-assess their learning to expand their learning. - Student occasionally contributes to class discussion	- Student will wait for the teacher to get help. - Student occasionally seeks help from another student. - Limited use of resources to get help
Ineffective	- Student cannot state what they are learning. - Student does not have "ownership" (does not use I statement) of the objective . - No objective posted so student unaware of the expectation.	- Student not aware of any way to assess their learning. - Student does not use any source within the room to assess their learning. - Student does not have a source for assessing their learning, that is rubric.	- Student compliant and does not contribute to expansion of the learning during large group instruction. - Lack of student participation or willingness to contributions to discussion	- Student waits for teacher to answer questions or concerns. - No effort is made by student to get help from classmate or classroom environment. - Student prefers to have teacher explanation.
Student Questions	- What are you learning today? - How will you learn? - How is what your learning important?	- Are you accomplishing your work? - How do you know you are doing well? - What questions do you ask yourself when you study?	- How will you plan to complete the assignment? - How does this assignment relate to the final product?	- Why do you seek help from your peers? - Can you resubmit your assignments? If so, how do you use the feedback you receive for future assignments?

© Dr. Pat Mitchell and Dr Mario C. Barbiere, March 2013. This rubric is copyrighted; permission to use must be obtained. This rubric and others are in Dr. Barbiere's text: *Teaching to the Learner's Brain: Instruction and Self Regulation*.

Appendix D

Rubric 4: Coaching Walkthrough Using the Learner's Brain Model

Coaching Walkthrough (CW) using the Learner's Brain Model (LBM)		
AREA	1=Ineffective; 2=Partially effective; 3=Effective; 4=Distinguished	
Principal's Focus:	Classroom #	
	# of students	
	Subject	
	Grade level(s)	
Readiness Stage for the Learner's Brain Model: Preparation for Instruction • Lesson plans closely align to curriculum • Common core state standards used • Differentiates activities to meet the needs of all learners planned • Activities planned for students who finish the assignment early. • Technology for instruction and learning planned • Pre-planned questions included in the lesson plan. • Closure planned *QSR Alignment: Leadership 1.5, 1.8; Effective Instruction 3.1, 3.2, 3.3, 3.5, 3.6; Curriculum, Assessment and Intervention 4.1, 4.2, 4.3, 4.5; Effective Use of Time 7.1 and 7.2* 1.5: principal ensures that a rigorous and coherent standards-based curriculum and aligned assessment system are implemented. 1.8: schedule aligned to school improvement plan 3.1: alignment of the objective to curriculum 3.2: teacher uses multiple instructional strategies to actively engage and meet students learning needs 3.3: teacher uses frequent checks for understanding (CFU) (used for lesson pacing) 3.5: teacher uses multiple sources of data, including formative of assessment, to differentiate instruction 4.1: school curriculum aligned to CCSS 4.2: verification of the "taught" curriculum – that is review of teacher lesson plans, use of standards in class 4.3: use of assessments to gauge instruction 4.5: intervention plan developed, monitored, and evaluated. 7.1: schedule designed to meet the needs of all students 7.2: master schedule meets the needs of students three years below	Review of Lesson Plans	Check if present
	Standards-based planning	
	Essential Question listed	
	Tiered lesson	
	Differentiated activities planned	
	Pre-planned questions	
	Plan for using technology	
	Closure planned	
	Comments: This component of the form looks at planning and instructional delivery. 1. Planning: social activities align to standards, differentiated aided instruction plan, and technology incorporated into the lesson. 2. Instructional delivery: is there appropriate pacing of the lesson as well as differentiation and for use of technology? 3. Is the essential question posted and referred back to students understand how their daily objectives addresses the essential question? 4. Does a teacher do constant checks for understanding to monitor and adjust the learning? 5. Do formative assessments guide instruction?	
Glows	**Grows**	

	Readiness Stage for the Learner's Brain Model: Lesson Objective/ Demonstration of Student Learning (DSL) • Lesson objective is posted • Objective written in student-friendly language • DSL posted • DSL written is in student-friendly terms *QSR Alignment : Effective Instruction 3.1* 3.1: Teacher ensures that student-friendly learning objectives are specific, measurable, attainable, realistic and timely, and are aligned to standards-based curriculum.					Check if present		
		Objective						
		DSL						
		Comments: 1. This component of the CW form is used to begin the process for self-regulation. 2. Students are informed of what they are expected to know and do (behavior) how they will be assessed (DSL). The "Bookends" of instruction: objective -beginning the curriculum; assessment – ends the process and informs teacher if the student achieved the objective.							

	Plan book _____ Posted = _____	Objective	(DSL)				
	Plan book						
	Posted						
	Verbs - RBT	Remember	Understand	Apply	Analyze	Evaluate	Create
	Verbs - Objective						
	Verbs - DOL						
4	Glows		Grows				

	Informational Stage for the Learner's Brain Model: Classroom Environment (Wall Walk) • Safe, organized, attractive, and designed to support learning • Procedures are in place to manage routines and materials • Posted or electronic student work samples reflect current and relevant learning objectives and exemplars • Current rubrics and meaningful written feedback is used to assess student work • Use of portfolios, journals, notebooks, or work folders (can be electronic) • Technology integration for instruction and learning *QSR Alignment: Leadership 1.3, 1.7; Climate and Culture 2.1; Effective Instruction 3.5, 3.6; Effective Use of Data 6.2 and 6.3* 1.3: principal uses data to work with staff to maintain an equitable learning environment 1.7: principal uses informal and formal observation data and ongoing student learning outcome data to	Displays of Learning	Check if present
		Rubrics & Exemplars	
		Meaningful Written Feedback	
		Routines & Labeling	
		Student Work Posted	
		Portfolios	
		Journals & Notebooks	
		Work Folders	
		Comments: In the classroom environment is established to help promote student self-regulation. Specifically: 1. Rubrics and exemplars are posted throughout the room for students to use to monitor their own learning. 2. Meaningful feedback is provided on student work. 3. Feedback is provided to clarify strength and to offer concrete specific information to the student for ways to improve. 4. Educational and informational charts for students to self-regulate. 5. The room is environmentally constructed to	

monitor and improve school-wide instructional practices and ensure the achievement of learning goals for all students (including SWD and ELLs) 2.1: school community supports a safe, orderly, and equitable learning environment 3.5: teacher uses multiple sources of data, including formative assessment, to differentiate instruction 3.6: teachers hold high expectations for all students academically and behaviorally as evidenced by their practice 6.2: multiple forms of data are presented to drive decisions for improving student achievement 6.3: process for analysis of assessment data tied to CCSS, which includes progress monitoring and evaluation	facilitate the students' self-regulation. 6. Routines and procedures are posted to provide a smooth transition within the classroom.
Glows	Grows
Input Stage for the Learner's Brain Model: Use of Data to Inform Instruction - Matches assessment method to assess proficiency of learning objective (rubrics, feedback devices, etc.) - Involves students in assessing their own learning during instruction - Conducts demonstrations of learning *QSR Alignment: Leadership 1.7; Effective Instruction 3.1, 3.3, 3.5; Curriculum, Assessment and Intervention 4.2, 4.3, 4.5; Effective Use of Data 6.2 and 6.3* 1.7: principal uses informal and formal observation data and ongoing student learning outcome data to monitor and improve school-wide instructional practices and ensure the achievement of learning goals for all students (including SWD and ELLs) 3.1: alignment of the objective to curriculum 3.2: teacher uses multiple instructional strategies to actively engage and meet students learning needs 3.3: teacher uses frequent CFU (used for lesson pacing) 3.5: teacher uses multiple sources of data, including formative assessment, to differentiate instruction 4.2: verification of the "taught" curriculum – that is review of teacher lesson plans, use of standards in class 4.3: use of assessments to gauge instruction	Comments: | Preparation Area	Check if present
Matches assessment method	
Involves students in assessing learning	
Conducts DOLs	| How is that the data used to inform instruction? 1. Does the teacher use checks for understanding monitor and adjust the lesson? 2. Do students self-assess throughout the lesson? 3. Are DOLs conducted? 4. Do students engage in self-regulation, that is referred to rubrics, exemplars or notes? 5. Data can be collected from the student during the instructional process or data can be collected as part of a summative process, that is DOLs, exit tickets, one-minute summary, got (what student understands), need (still need to know), or other types of assessments. 6. Is meaningful feedback provided so that it is user-friendly, specific, personalized, and actionable?

	4.5: intervention plan developed, monitored, and evaluated 6.2: multiple forms of data are presented to drive decisions for improving student achievement 6.3: process for analysis of assessment data tied to CCSS, which includes progress monitoring and evaluation	Rating
	Glows	Grows
5	**Input Stage of the Learner's Brain Model: Student Engagement (Instruction)** • Engages students within one minute of bell • Engages all students in the lesson • Uses smooth transitions and provides closure • Selects multiple instructional strategies that maintain focus and engage students • Solicits multiple responses from all students to check for understanding • Lesson focus on rigorous content, relevant to the grade level *QSR Alignment: Effective Instruction 3.2, 3.3, and 3.6* 3.2: teacher uses multiple instructional strategies to actively engage and meet students learning needs 3.3: teacher uses frequent CFU (used for lesson pacing) 3.6: teachers hold high expectations for all students academically and behaviorally as evidenced by their practice	Number of students Number of students following lesson/observing teacher Number of students actively responding to teacher Comments: The key to student engagement is: the more the teacher talks and the students listen, the lower the teacher rating. The more the student does, the higher, the teacher is rated. A critical factor in determining student engagement what the students are doing and not if students are compliant. Important considerations are: 1. Students engaging in cooperative activities 2. Are multiple learning styles used throughout the instructional delivery? 3. Does the teacher check for understanding and monitor the lesson accordingly? 4. Do students also regulate the learning? 5. What are the students doing as a result of what the teacher has said or done? 6. How do students initially, adapt, promote activities and assignments? Rating
	Glows	Grows

Effective Instruction/Student Communication • Bloom's Taxonomy Level • Higher-Order Thinking and Questioning • Students able to communicate what they know and take risks in ways that include thoughtful analysis of new information, personal perspectives, and imagination. • Circulates during instruction and activities; monitors student progress (proximity, journals, student response) • Interactions that are positive and respectful *QSR Alignment: Leadership 1.5; Effective Instruction 3.1 and 3.3* 1.5: principal ensures rigorous and coherent standards-based curriculum and aligned assessment system 3.1: alignment of the objective to curriculum 3.3: teacher uses frequent CFU (used for lesson pacing)	Level of Communication	Check if observed
	Remember	
	Understand	
	Apply	
	Analyze	
	Evaluate	
	Create	

Do students discriminate, deconstruct, judge, and identify inconsistencies, and use criteria to put elements together to form a coherent or functional whole. (Higher level on Bloom's Revised Taxonomy BRT).

Higher order questions promote cognitive stimulation and discussion, not recitation.

Questions are divergent and open-ended.

Glows	Grows

Student Interviews (Students are selected at random.) • What are you working on? Or: What are you doing? • How do you assess your own learning? Are you called upon to respond for understanding? • What do you do when you need help or assistance? *QSR Alignment: Leadership 1.4, 1.5; Effective Instruction 3.1, 3.2, and 3.6* 1.4: The principal communicates high expectations to staff, students, and families, and supports students to achieve them.	Total # of students interviewed	
	Question	# answering question
	What are you working on?	
	How do you assess your own learning?	
	Are you called upon to respond for understanding?	
	What do you do when you need help or assistance?	

Comments:

When students are asked what are they leasrning today, they are able to articulate the objectives and its relationship to the overall goal.

Students self-regulate and monitor their own work.

Students seek help for assistance from their classmates or from other sources prior to going to the teacher as they engage in the process of self-regulation.

Student participation is not an option as the teacher uses random sources methods to ensure student participation.

Comments

Overall Glows

Overall Grows

Suggestions

Follow up

Index

Note. Page references for figures and tables are italicized.

accommodations, 16–17, 49
activities: checking for understanding, 46–47; closing, 67–70; create a jingle, 67; exit ticket, 8; fishbowl, 67; infomercial, 67; large group, 42; movie review, 68; small groups, 19, 43–44; throwing the ball, 67; "What Am I?", 67
analogies, 27
asking why questions, 34
assessments, 17, 33–57; action theory for, 7; auditory learners, 51; being overt, 50; conventional thinking of, 35; effectiveness, 51–52; formative, 7–8; as an instructional strategy, 34; for learning, 36–40; mind-set shift, 52–53; overview, 33–34; self-regulation and, 35–36; tactile learners, 51; teachers view on, 7; visual learners, 50. *See also* checking for understanding; formative assessments
attribution theory, 53–54
auditory learners, assessment of, 51

Black, Paul, 51–52
bodily kinesthetic intelligence, 16, 48

Castle, Christine, 36
chain map, 19
chart: KWL/KWHL, 15; organizational, 18–19. *See also* map
checking for understanding, 14–15; activities promoting, 46–47; examples of, *45–46*; pitfalls, 23–24
Classroom Instruction That Works: Research Based Strategies for Increasing Student Achievement (Marzano, Pickering, and Pollock), 20–21
closing activities, 67–70; create a jingle, 67; exit ticket, 8; fishbowl, 67; infomercial, 67; movie review, 68; throwing the ball, 67; "What Am I?", 67
closure: activities, 67–70; based on learning styles, *69–70*; benefits, 65–66; concept of, 63; consolidation, 65; feedback and, 66; overt/covert, *68–69*; procedural, 65; psychological process of, 63; research, 63–64; review *vs.*, 62–63
cognitive strategies, 54–57. *See also* distributed practice; massed practice

collaborative reflective environment, 83–84
competency, 20
concept map, 18
consolidation closure, 65
consolidation for closure, 17, 50, 61–70; backward framing to, 64; process, 64–65; sunny point/cloudy point, 8–9
cooperative groups, 19
cooperative learning, 19
covert closure, 68–69. See also overt closure
cramming, 55; spacing vs., 55–56. See also massed practice
create a jingle, as closing activity, 67
critical point, 29
cross-curricular questions, 40
curricula: driving instructional delivery, 7

Danielson, Charlotte, 77, 80
demonstration of student learning (DSL), 42
Dewey, John, 76, 82
differentiated instruction, 105–13
distributed practice: concept, 22; example of, 22–23; massed practice vs., 54; pre-home learning questions, 23; strategies for, 56. See also interleaving; spacing vs. cramming
DSL. See demonstration of student learning

elaborative interrogation, 57
empowerment, teachers, 83
engagement, 28–29
exit ticket activity, 8
"Experience and Education" (Dewey), 76

feedback, 15; closure offering, 66; practice, 20; quizzes, 57; timely and constructive, 53
fishbowl closing activity, 67
formative assessments, 7–8, 49; effectiveness of, 51–52; strategies for, 57. See also assessments

four-square template, 13, 14, 15
Frog and Toad Are Friends, 16

Gestalt psychology, 63
group activities: large, 42; small, 19, 43–44
group reflection, 83–84
guided practice, 17, *21*; of small groups, 44–47

healthful living, sample lesson, 37–40
healthy heart, sample lesson on, 37–40
heart. See healthy heart, sample lesson on
hierarchy map, 18–19
home learning, 22; generalizations about, 29; promoting, 29; research on, 29–30
homework: assignments, 22; feedback from, 20; instructional purposes, 30; scholastic skills development, 30; student achievement and, 30
Horn, Sandra, 51

IEP. See Individualized Education Plans
independent practice, 17–19, 23–27, 50; checking for understanding pitfalls, 23–24; specific strategies to use, 24–27
Individualized Education Plans (IEP), 14
infomercial, as closing activity, 67
instructional delivery, *18*, 18–19
instructional input, 13–14, 42
intelligence. See multiple intelligences
interleaving, 54–55; example of, 55; strategies to use for, 56–57
interpersonal intelligence, 16, 49
intrapersonal intelligence, 16, 49

KWL/KWHL chart, 15

language arts, 10–12. See also writing
large group activity, 42
learning, assessments for, 36–40

learning styles: addressing, 42; assessment modalities, 50–51
lesson development, teacher reflection and, 85
lesson planning. *See* sample lesson
linguistic intelligence, 15, 48
logical–mathematical intelligence, 15, 48
long-term learning. *See* distributed practice

manipulatives, 26
map: chain, 19; concept, 18; hierarchy, 18–19. *See also* chart
Marshall, Kim, 79–80
Marzano, R. J., 20–21, 22, 63
massed practice, 54; concept, 22; distributed practice *vs.*, 54; example of, 22–23; pre-home learning questions, 23; strategies for, 56. *See also* cramming
math, sample lesson, 105–13
mental imagery, 18
mind-set shift, 52–53
modeling, 14, 42
monitoring, 17; self-regulation and, 35–36; of small groups, 44–47
movie review, as closing activity, 68
multiple intelligences, 15–19; accommodations, 16–17, 49; assessments, 17, 49; bodily kinesthetic, 16, 48; consolidation for closure, 17, 50; guided practice and monitoring, 17; independent practice, 17–19, 50; interpersonal, 16, 49; intrapersonal, 16, 49; linguistic, 15, 48; logical–mathematical, 15, 48; musical, 15–16, 48; naturalist, 16, 49; spatial–visual, 16, 48–49
musical intelligence, 15–16, 48

naturalist intelligence, 16, 49
nonlinguistic representations, 18

open-ended questions, 86–87
organizational chart, 18–19

overt closure, *68–69*. *See also* covert closure

persuasive writing, lesson planning, 89–105. *See also* writing
Pickering, D., 20–21, 22, 63
planning: critical questions for, 7
Pollock, Jane E., 20–21, 22, 63
practice, 19–22; competency, 20; conditions to be considered for, 20; feedback, 20; perfect, 19–20; self-regulated learning (SRL), 20
primacy-recency, 20
procedural closure, 65
professional development, teacher reflection and, 84
Pyc, M. A., 54

questions: asking why, 34; promoting stimulation of prior knowledge, 39
quizzes, 57. *See also* assessments

Readiness Set, 6, 9, 12–13, 25, 26, 39–47; addressing learning styles, 42; checking for understanding, 44, 45–47; closing activities, 47; DSL, 42; formative assessment, 44; guided practice and monitoring of small groups, 44–46, *45–46*; instructional input, 42; large group activity, 42; sense and meaning activity, 41; small group activity, 43–44
reference materials, 14
reflection, 73–87; concept, 76, 82; overview, 73–74; process of, 80–85; reasons given for not doing, 79; as sports coach, 74; student, 85–87; as teachers, 74; testimony, 74–75. *See also* student reflection; teacher reflection
reflection after, 77, *78*
reflection before, 77, *78*
reflection during, 77–78, *78*
reinforce effort, 27–28

review *vs.* closure, 62–63
Roediger, H. L., 54

sample lesson, 89–113; differentiated instruction, 105–13; healthful living and healthy heart, 37–40; math, 105–13; persuasive writing, 89–105; science, 9–10
Sanders, William, 51
school-dependent learning: concept, 52; shift towards school-dependent learning, 52
science, sample lesson, 9–10
self-dependent learning: concept, 52; mind-set shift toward, 52–53
self-management, 87
self-monitoring interventions, 87
self-regulated learning (SRL), 20; mind-set shift toward, 52–53
self-regulation: classroom environment and, 35; monitoring for, 35–36; promoting, 35–36; SRL strategies and, 35; using assessments for, 35–36
sense and meaning making, 23, 24, 28, 41
short-term learning. *See* massed practice
small groups: activities, 19, 43–44; guided practice and monitoring of, 44–47
spacing *vs.* cramming, 55–56
spatial–visual intelligence, 16, 48–49
spider model, 18
sports coach, reflection as, 74
stories, 27; four-square templates, 14; writing, 14, 15
student reflection, 74, 85–87; open-ended questions, 86–87; questions promoting, 86; reasons being important, 85–86
student self-explanation, 57

tactile learners, assessment of, 51
TBM (Two before Me), 10, 36
teacher evaluation, reflection and, 77, 79–80
Teacher Evaluation Rubric (Marshall), 79–80
teacher reflection, 78–80; background, 75–78; dilemma and outcomes, 75–76; evaluation and, 77, 79–80; group reflection, 83–84; learning from experience, 80–81; lesson development and, 85; lesson study, 81; professional development and, 84; promoting, 81; reflection after, 77, *78*; reflection before, 77, *78*; reflection during, 77–78, *78*; rubrics for, 77
teachers: dilemma, 75; empowerment, 83; primary responsibility of, 76; reasons given for not doing reflection, 79
tests. *See* assessments
throwing the ball, as closing activity, 67

Uilian, Dylan, 51–52
understanding, checking for. *See* checking for understanding

visual learners, assessment of, 50
visual representations, 25, 26

websites, 40
Weird Friends, Unlikely Allies in the Animal Kingdom, 13, 16
"What Am I?", as closing activity, 67
why questions, 34
Wright, S. Paul, 51
writing, 10–12; brainstorming, 15; forms, audiences, and purposes, 11; lesson planning, 89–105; mechanics, spelling, handwriting, 11; as a process, 10–11; as a product, 11; reference materials for, 14; word choice, 12

About the Author

Dr. Mario C. Barbiere has administrative experience at all district levels and has also taught college classes as an associate professor. He has extensive work experience in school turnaround beginning with serving as Network Turnaround Officer (NTO) for two inner-city schools that had been low performing. Working with the principal and teachers, both schools doubled their test scores in one year and became higher-achieving schools. After that, Dr. Barbiere was executive director for Regional Achievement Center, Region 5, which was created to work with low-performing schools or schools with an achievement gap. Under the Every Student Succeed Act, the Regional Achievement Centers were identified as Comprehensive Support and Improvement Teams and Dr. Barbiere was the regional executive director.

His doctoral studies were in brain research and lesson design. The research developed interest in instructional delivery and student self-regulation.

Having the opportunity to work in a variety of schools, Dr. Barbiere is passionate about teaching and student empowerment so students are empowered and self-dependent and not teacher- or school-dependent.

CPSIA information can be obtained
at www.ICGtesting.com
Printed in the USA
LVHW031133271019
635473LV00002B/376/P